"This beautiful book takes us way beyond weight loss to a new appreciation of total health, inner and outer beauty, and a loving truce with food."

—**John Robbins**, author of *Diet for a New America*

"If you have been seeking a new relationship—with food, with your body, with life—Victoria Moran's book is the magic ingredient you need. It is a recipe for sane, safe eating..."

—**Michael Klaper**, M.D., Scientific director of EarthSave and author of *Vegan Nutrition: Pure and Simple*

"Courageous, forthright, warm, and informative. I give it my highest recommendation... *The Love-Powered Diet* has affected my life."

—**Benjamin Shield**, Ph.D., co-author of *Handbook for the Soul* and *Handbook for the Heart*

"In *The Love-Powered Diet* you'll learn ways to make immediate changes in your attitude and diet that will have a profound effect on your self-esteem, health, and life. If you want to look younger, lose weight for good, prevent disease, reclaim your life, or just feel radiantly healthy, this superb, practical guide was written just for you."

—**Susan Smith Jones, Ph.D.**, author of *Choose Radiant Health and Happiness*

"While making us salivate for the crunch and fun of healthy eating, Victoria delivers the best message of all, that keeping off lost weight requires maintenance of a fit spiritual condition. Such an enjoyable romp into understanding what foods work and why."

—**Judi Hollis**, author of *Fat is a Family Affair*

THE
LOVE-POWERED
DIET

Eating for Freedom, Health, and Joy

VICTORIA MORAN

LANTERN BOOKS • NEW YORK
A DIVISION OF BOOKLIGHT INC.

2009
Lantern Books
128 Second Place, Garden Suite
Brooklyn, NY 11231

Printed in the United States

Cover designer: Stefan Killen (stefankillendesign.com)
Cover photo: David Rodgers (davidrodgersphotography.com)

The Twelve Steps and brief excerpts are reprinted with permission of Alcoholics Anonymous World Services, Inc. Permission to reprint this material does not mean that AA has reviewed or approved the contents of this publication, nor that AA agrees with the views expressed herein. AA is a program of recovery from alcoholism—use of these excerpts in connection with programs and activities that are patterned after AA, but that address other problems, does not imply otherwise.

Notice: This book is intended as a reference volume only, not as a medical manual. The information given here is designed to help you make informed decisions about your health. It's not intended as a substitute for any treatment that may have been prescribed or recommendations given by your health care provider. If you suspect that you have a medical problem, we urge you to seek competent medical help.

Library of Congress Cataloging-in-Publication Data

Moran, Victoria, 1950-
 The love-powered diet : eating for freedom, health, and joy / by Victoria Moran.
   p. cm.
 ISBN-13: 978-1-59056-117-1 (alk. paper)
 ISBN-10: 1-59056-117-1 (alk. paper)
 1. Weight loss--Religious aspects. 2. Weight loss--Psychological aspects. 3. Self-esteem. 4. Self-acceptance.
5. Love. 6. Compulsive eating--Religious aspects. I. Title.
 RM222.2.M568 2009
 613.2'5--dc22
                        2008032827

To My Daughter

Thank you for your patience in sharing more than two years of your childhood with this project in its original form, and for your continuing inspiration. For any good this book does, at least half the credit is yours.

CONTENTS

ACKNOWLEDGMENTS

I wish to thank Martin Rowe and everyone at Lantern Books for their decision to publish this new edition of *The Love-Powered Diet*; my friend Patti Breitman, agent for this book once again; and everyone who kept saying: "That book was before its time. It needs to be published again." Among these staunch supporters are Karen Kelly, editor of the second edition (its title then was *Love Yourself Thin*); John Pierre, a Chicago personal trainer and lifestyle coach who uses the book with his clients; and my longtime friend Lane Martin who has championed *The Love-Powered Diet* from its beginnings.

I also owe a special debt of gratitude to another great friend and wordsmith in her own right, Elizabeth Cutting, who brought this book in its previous form to a publisher-ready manuscript. Thanks also go to the professionals who offered their nutritional expertise: George Eisman, RD, Suzanne Havala-Hobbs, MS, RD, MPH, and Michael Klaper, MD; and to Mary Max for her generous website recommendations and for the "Veggie by Brand" sidebar in Chapter Eight.

Finally, I extend my appreciation to the many individuals who filled out questionnaires concerning their recovery from food addiction; the many writers, teachers, and mentors in the world of compassionate living and plant-based dining; the hundreds of recovering people who have guided and educated me over the years; and to Alcoholics Anonymous and Overeaters Anonymous for the wisdom of the Twelve Steps.

FOREWORD TO THE THIRD EDITION

*T*he *Love-Powered Diet* was first published in 1992 by New World Library. In 1997, it was revised and re-released by Daybreak, an imprint of Rodale Books, with the title *Love Yourself Thin*. When I wrote the original text, the now accepted notion that overeating could be a disease or addiction similar to alcoholism, drug addiction, or compulsive gambling was widely discounted, and most people believed that "going on a diet" would solve the problem.

We've come a long way. There's more understanding today of the kind of eating that's done to fill an inner void, and that the same kind of recovery process shown by time to work on all manner of addictions can address food addiction as well. The scientific studies about the health benefits of a plant-based diet were just beginning to surface when I wrote *The Love-Powered Diet* in its first version and they have continued to mount. There's now irrefutable research showing that fruits, vegetables, legumes, and whole grains are the foods of choice for good health, long life, and maintaining proper weight without the agony of dieting.

There's one thing that hasn't changed in all this time, however: I've continued to be blessed with freedom from compulsive overeating. I continue living in a fit, healthy body, and being free from worry about how much I weigh or what I'm going to eat. This is a gift that I trust you, too, will receive as you read this book and do what it says.

The Love-Powered Diet addresses a dual dilemma: the addictive nature of overeating and the nutritional shortfalls of the standard American diet. It offers solutions for both. I see the benefits of this way of living and eating every day in friends, colleagues, clients in my life-coaching practice, and in my own evolving experience. Some readers of this book will relate to the spiritual part of the process and grab on to Twelve-Step recovery like a life raft. They'll use the principles on their own or join Overeaters Anonymous and find hope there that they never knew existed.

Others will take to the dietary principles, a compassionate way of eating that allows for weight loss and maintenance without deprivation, dieting, weighing and measuring every morsel, and worrying that the weight will come back. Those who find a way to apply both strands of love-powered living—spiritual and dietary—to their own circumstances will benefit most.

I wish you peace, health, and happiness, and an open heart.

—**Victoria Moran**
Woodstock, New York
June 2008

AUTHOR'S NOTE

The premise of *The Love-Powered Diet* is simple. It's one idea with two parts:

(1) Inner awareness of unconditional love can make profound changes in a person's life.

(2) Inner change includes the ability to make positive, loving food choices.

This book is especially addressed to food addicts —that is, any person of any body size who's engaged in a longstanding battle with a knife and fork. Its principles can, however, help anyone eat more healthfully and live more happily.

The format of the Twelve Steps, originally developed by Alcoholics Anonymous, is used in this book. These steps aren't the only way to bring about a spiritual awakening powerful enough to change one's life and behavior, but they have had unparalleled success in helping people with a wide range of dependencies, including alcohol, drugs, unhealthy relationships, and compulsive eating. There is no official or unofficial connection between this book and any Twelve Step organization.

The loving food choices referred to involve selecting natural foods from the plant kingdom that promote physical health and discourage overeating. Choosing these foods expresses love not only to oneself but to nonhuman animals and the environment. Connecting this way of eating to a Twelve Step lifestyle is my idea, and Overeaters Anonymous, the largest and most visible Twelve Step program for people with food issues, does not endorse this or any other particular dietary choice.

The spiritual and physical aspects presented in this book are, however, two parts of a single whole. There are many people who have overcome eating disorders by approaching food differently than I suggest, and there are people who have lost weight and kept it off simply by switching to a plant-based diet. Nevertheless, linking the two creates a winning combination. In fact, one can lead to the other. People who deepen their spiritual lives often evolve toward a gentler, more natural diet. Conversely, those who discover natural foods, particularly men and women who become vegetarians or vegans, are often led to explore their spiritual natures.

Recognizing that spirituality is an emotionally charged subject for many people, I've done my best to keep my vocabulary and references acceptable both to people who are traditionally religious and those who are not. If any references in this book make you uncomfortable, feel free to substitute another word or phrase, such as "Spirit" for "God." You do not have to change your beliefs about religion or the afterlife to draw upon the love already inside you to make this a life of freedom and joy.

INTRODUCTION

This is your fairy godmother speaking: You can have a body you think is gorgeous—not just for the ball, but forever. You can go to sleep at night without hating yourself for what you ate during the day, and you'll never again need to count calories or carbohydrates, grams of fat or ounces of food. You only need to count yourself lucky for having discovered a new way of seeing and doing things.

OK, so I'm not your fairy godmother. I'm another person just like you with a food problem that took me around the block so many times I could have passed as a meter reader. I cannot zap you with a magic wand. You'll just *think* I did once you discover within yourself a source of power to change your eating and your life—one that's more effective than a regiment of fairy godmothers marching in formation. This is the power of love. Don't be put off by an overused word. It's an extremely underused resource.

You know how being *in love* transforms the way people look and feel, and how loving someone or something can give a person a sense of purpose and power. There's more than one story about a small woman lifting an automobile off her child trapped beneath it. There's also abundant evidence of the crucial role that love plays in healing. Physicians such as Bernie Siegel, Larry Dossey, and Deepak Chopra have documented how loving oneself and others can mean the difference between getting well and giving up. When patients open themselves to love as an active energy in its own right, they can experience changes in their own bodies and emotions that appear miraculous. Some think of this as divine love, others as the synchronizing force that keeps electrons whirling about the nucleus of every atom. It works either way.

This love can revolutionize your relationship with food because the love already inside you is not only strengthening, it's *filling*. If you have a history of overeating and being overweight—or its flip side of chronic dieting, bulimia, or over-exercising—you may have already realized that you're not eating to fill your stomach. You're eating to fill a gash in your soul.

There isn't enough food on Earth to fill that inner void, and there aren't enough friends, lovers, or children, houses, cars, or stock certificates, clothes, compliments, or accomplishments to fill it either. Nevertheless, when you connect with the love inside you, a comfortable sense of *enoughness* begins to emerge. The dictionary claims that "enoughness" isn't a word, but without it, you and food will always be at war.

You win this battle when you give up the fight. Attach your willpower to the nearest white flag and let love take over. That's when you'll understand that you are enough. You are attractive enough. You are lovable enough. And for this day, the most important one there is, you are thin enough, too. When I use the word *thin*, I don't mean model-thin or athlete-thin or adolescent-thin. I mean feeling comfortable with your body and proud to walk around in it. Thin, as used in this book, means having a body that serves you well so you can live freely without wishing you weighed less.

Do you know what will happen when you comprehend—not just with your head but with your heart and your spirit—that you're indeed thin enough for the day at hand, that you're truly attractive and lovable? You'll treat yourself as someone who's all those things. For starters, you'll eat a like a thin, attractive, lovable person does. When I was fighting food with the vigor of a fresh Marine recruit, a wise old fellow told me that I was putting the cart before the horse in trying to eat less than I wanted and to exercise more. He said that it works the other way around, that people who are healthy automatically do healthy things.

Every concerned and loving action you take shows the love-empowerment working in your life. Using a cloth bag instead of plastic is like making yourself a couple of baked potatoes instead of tearing into a bag of chips. Both show you care, and it's pretty difficult to practice genuine caring and addictive behavior at the same time.

Goodness knows, I was an authority on healthy things. I'd been writing articles about health, fitness, and beauty since I was nineteen. I read, researched, and wrote, keeping abreast of the latest trends in diet, nutrition, exercise, and behavior modification. I interviewed experts and passed their findings along. I'd accumulated so much information that my head ached, but I was trapped in a binge/diet cycle so insidious that most of the time, my heart ached, too.

It was embarrassing enough to go from fat to thin and back again like a human accordion. In addition to seeing myself as a diet failure, I saw myself as a phony. The words I wrote were true based on the knowledge available at the time, but I wasn't able to put them into practice. Like a marriage counselor going through his fifth divorce, my work and my life were sorely fragmented.

Fragmentation—fragmented lives in a fragmented society—is a component most of the time when eating is out of balance. The love-powered approach meets fragmentation with integration because pure, essential love is an integrating force. It doesn't foster bits and pieces. Love will not only make a difference in what you eat and the amount of exercise you get but it will also enhance the way you feel about your body. The integrating power of love can bring all your parts into a functioning whole. When it infuses the way you eat and the way you live, your body will definitely show results, but so will every other aspect of your life. Nothing less than that can bring about changes that last.

When love fills your emptiness and integrates your fragmented factions, you'll no longer need a closet filled with clothes that range in size from 2 to triple-X. You won't need to be a person who starts every Monday with a dismal diet that's tossed aside by Tuesday afternoon. You can stop spending your money on every pill, potion, and promise that comes around. The kind of love I'm talking about keeps its promises a day at a time, as surely as the sun brings light in the morning. Without that, weight loss is destined to be temporary. You know that's as true as an oath in court because you've lost weight before. You'd be better off keeping the body you have right now and learning to cherish it than to have one more raving success with a diet, then blow the lid off it and despise yourself. Those episodes erode the spirit. You deserve the chance to leave them behind for good.

The only way I know to bring destructive eating to a screeching halt and keep it there on a daily basis is to let love take care of it. I not only tried the other ways, I wrote articles about them. There were plenty of good ideas in those approaches. Many were sane and logical, devised by intelligent, caring people, but the power to make them work for me wasn't in them. They presented valid facts about nutrition or working out or "thinking thin," but these facts were as useless to me as one perfectly decent battery in a flashlight that needs two.

The love-powered approach is different because it works on both perspective and practice. On an inner level, it means trading willpower for love's power. In practical application, it means living and eating in love-inspired fashion. The foods you'll prefer will be those that express love—to your physical self, to all livingkind, and to the planet that provides our food in the first place. You won't be dieting. It's known now that that kind of regimentation can't realistically be imposed on natural processes, and that responding to hunger is as natural to us as blinking or breathing. Instead of dieting, you'll be choosing to care for yourself and those around you as you make your selections at the supermarket or from the menu.

Because you're worth the best, your way of eating will reflect the low-fat, high-fiber, high-complex-carbohydrate recommendations of the American Heart Association, the American Cancer Society, and the overwhelming majority of human nutrition studies of the past forty years. In fact, it will epitomize these recommendations. And luscious fruits, colorful vegetables, hearty whole grains, and protein-rich legumes satisfy hunger while they discourage cravings. With a loving attitude and these foods as the staples in your kitchen, you really *can* eat all you want because what you want will finally be what you need. Weight loss and maintenance will proceed spontaneously without undue attention. You can stop watching your weight and start seeing the beauty that's in and around you. In this way, love works in you to make your life better and through you to make your world better.

There's an old maxim that says, "He who lives for himself alone lives for the meanest mortal known." Those who eat for themselves alone are in something of the same category. One of the reasons why diets so often fail is that, instead of bringing you into the stream of life, they set you apart from it—off somewhere with your blender and your portion scale and your food diary. With the love-powered approach, being part of life is part of the solution.

Is this going to be complicated? No, it's deceptively simple. Will it be easy? Not all the time, but living this way is, at its toughest, easier than trying to convince yourself that the ice cream in your shopping cart is for the family, when you know that your husband is out of town and both your kids are allergic to dairy. Probably the most difficult thing you'll have to grapple with is giving up the fight. You may feel as if you've gone AWOL, but believe me: with love as your commander-in-chief you'll be honorably discharged from active combat. You'll be able to harmonize an inner awareness of love with loving outward actions—food choices included.

This harmony is essential for durable change, whether you want to overcome chronic binge eating, do away with an annoying ten pounds, stop dieting for the first time since puberty, or simply eat a little more healthfully than you do now. Life without the dual plagues of compulsive eating and fanatical weight control is precious indeed. Health of body and peace of mind are also priceless commodities. To help you toward these, love yourself to a new relationship with food; love yourself to a new appreciation for yourself and your body; and love yourself thin without forcing yourself there.

CHAPTER ONE

MY STORY
(AND FOOD AS A FIX)

I was a fat little girl in a fat-phobic family There was a diet for me taped to the refrigerator and I only got a milkshake when I was sick. Years later I had a cold and my boyfriend brought me a French vanilla shake. I married him. You see, my father had been a physician who had gradually turned his practice from ear, nose, and throat to fat, flab, and cellulite. My mother managed "reducing salons"—anemic precursors to the modern health club—with adipose-jiggling machines and the promise of effortless weight loss. I knew early on that my plumpness was not pleasing and that I was bad for business.

It wasn't that I didn't want to be good and stick to my diet. I knew that there were starving children who didn't even have grapefruit and grilled halibut, but the notion of restricting what I ate was terrifying. It meant giving up the sublime security that came from an illicit cookie or a bag of trail mix (that's healthy, right?). When I was eating, I felt safe, content, and loved. Once the food was gone, so was the feeling. Like everyone else, I needed food to sustain life, but I also needed it to face life. I didn't know it then, but I was hooked. Food was my fix.

When I was thirteen, I discovered the flipside of my addiction: the high of being thin. I'd been sick and wasn't able to eat for a couple of weeks. Once I got out of bed, I weighed myself: 111 pounds. I had bones. They were wonderful. I was wonderful. I bought a gorgeous green satin dress with puffy sleeves and a dropped waist and a flippy little skirt. I was awed by own reflection in the mirror. I thought I looked like the models in the teen magazines. I could have died in peace at that moment. I was finally OK.

I never got to go anywhere in that green satin dress, however. I was back to 140 pounds in little over a month, and I felt for the first time "pitiful and incomprehensible demoralization"—the phrase the book *Alcoholics Anonymous* uses to describe the state of an alcoholic who had once gained some control and then lost it again. I never drank, but the phrase fit.

I didn't realize then that, as with the alcoholic, control wasn't the point. I was ill when it came to food, and I could no more control my eating than I could "control" the healing of a broken leg. That's why all my stalwart attempts at managing my eating ended as dismal failures.

One of these came for me at age twenty when I lost weight with a popular commercial weight-loss system. When I reached the prescribed "goal weight," I was afraid to go off the diet and got down to the absurdly low weight of 98 pounds. Unlike an anorexic who would have kept on losing, I took my two-digit reading on the scale as evidence that I'd broken the thin barrier. I was cured. I bought a pound of roasted cashews, ate them all on the bus ride home. I kept this up and gained twenty pounds in sixty days.

Had I been sane, I'd have realized that that put me at my ideal weight, but instead I saw myself on an unstoppable course that would take me further and further up in poundage and down in self-esteem. "Pitiful and incomprehensible demoralization" combined with such hatred for my eventually inflated body that I refused to be seen by anyone who knew me. I quit my job and moved to Chicago where I planned to hide, diet, and return at some future date in triumphant thinness.

While in Chicago, I learned to fast, perfecting two-week stints on water only and doing several short juice fasts as well. My physical self shrank obediently every time, but I was so ravenous after each of these Gandhian intervals that, after eighteen months on a starve–binge cycle, the final tally was a weight gain of over fifty pounds. After that, I stayed away from scales.

It took months for my ability to diet to resurface. I was inspired by my boyfriend's taking off for the West Coast, maybe to come back, maybe not. Hurt and anger mobilized my resolve: I'd get thin and beautiful and show him what he'd left behind. I lost weight and he proposed, but neither of us realized that, heavy or slim, I was a food addict.

The façade started to crack with little weight gains here and there. They were frightening, and I felt I couldn't trust myself around a refrigerator while subject to any of the ordinary pressures of life—work, my roommate, my cat. The answer: fat farms. I took a week in Texas the first time, then two in Florida. It was becoming an expensive habit, so I started checking myself into nice local hotels to diet or fast and use their health club facilities. It worked well for a while, but as I needed to go more frequently, cost again became an issue.

I looked for cheaper and cheaper hotels. The last was a past-its-prime hostelry at the tawdry end of downtown. It had a phone book minus the Yellow Pages and a Gideon Bible lacking most of the New Testament. The carpet had been burned in spots by a careless smoker and the television was chained to the wall. "I'm in a bona fide flophouse," I told myself. "And I got here with a fork." I cried most of the night because I knew I'd become the equivalent of a gutter drunk, but if I told anyone that, they'd laugh and tell me to push myself away from the table.

It was becoming obvious that I had a problem that went beyond calories in and calories burned, so I sought help from various therapists and counselors who pointed out numerous reasons why I ate the way I did. The list was impressive:

- I'd had a digestive disorder as an infant, so I carried with me a primal fear of starvation
- My parents' professions had set me up for an eating disorder, and my staying overweight was an unconscious ploy to demand their unconditional love
- Since I'd been a heavy kid, I had a greater number of fat cells than people who had gained weight in adulthood and simply enlarged the ones they had; all those greedy lipid cells were crying out to be fed
- I had, according to one unconventional psychologist, died of hunger in a past life and was trying to make up for it in this one.

Some Things Food Addicts May Do

. . . .

- Hide food

- Sneak food

- Go on diets, usually on Mondays

- Make promises, vows, and deals with themselves, others, and God about eating less and losing weight

- Lie to themselves, others, and God

- Avoid scales or weigh themselves compulsively

- Dissociate from their bodies—live from the neck up

- Put off living—shopping, swimming, vacationing, making love—until weight is lost

- Detest physical exercise or become addicted to exercise (but may still detest it)

- Feel unattractive or conditionally attractive based on a scale number or clothing size

- Hate fat people (or hate thin people)

- Have special binge foods as drugs of choice (chocolate, sweets, salty snacks, cheese, and rich, creamy foods are favorites) but could binge on almost anything in a pinch

- Vomit after a binge or even after a moderate meal or snack (bulimia)

- Eat others' leftovers, unthawed frozen foods, or nonfoods (e.g., the paper from around a muffin, used tea bags, chewing gum)

- Diet successfully for a time, then gain back as much or more weight than was lost (the ability to diet eventually ceases altogether)

- Find it easier to fast than to eat moderately

- Push food on other people, especially when depriving themselves

- Cook and bake—though in later stages of the disease, these may fall aside in favor of readymade, instant-gratification items

- Please people, be *sweet*

- Make jokes, be *jolly*

- Be defensive, feel put upon, take up the cause of "fat lib"

- Deal inappropriately with anger, either denying ("stuffing") it or having attacks of rage, usually toward someone powerless, such as a child or companion animal

- Switch compulsions, such as giving up food for a time and becoming addicted to drugs, sex, working, or spending

I was grateful to learn all these fascinating hypotheses about my behavior. Unfortunately, being so enlightened didn't change a thing. The solution, if there was to be one, had to come in another way. And it did. I didn't outgrow my food addiction, I don't have any more willpower than I ever did, and I haven't had broiled halibut in decades. Nevertheless, I didn't eat for a fix today and I didn't obsess over the size and shape of my body. As a practicing food addict, I was helpless, but I was never hopeless. Neither are you.

Patterns

You may eat for a fix in many of the ways that I did. The pattern may have started early in life or when you got married or after you were divorced. You may trace it to a pregnancy or the loss of someone you loved, or it may have come upon you subtly and gradually. You may eat enormous meals or snack all day and not even remember when you had your last real breakfast, lunch, or dinner. You may only eat unreasonably when it comes to chocolate or other sweets, or salty, crunchy snacks. Perhaps you eat sparingly around other people and binge on the sly so no one can understand why you can't lose weight. ("She eats like a bird," you've heard them say, "but she's as big as a house.")

On the other hand, you may be enviably slim and only you know that you stay that way by throwing up every day or that your preoccupation with fitness long ago shifted from a healthy habit to a tyrannical compulsion. You could be eating quite reasonably and looking fine but you feel fat, berate yourself, and believe that if only you had a perfect body, you could live a perfect life. Maybe you're so devastated by the addiction that you avoid people as much as you can and hardly bother to wash the one outfit that you can still wear. More likely, though, you seem to function flawlessly and keep on top of everything except for a "little problem with eating." It's also possible that you don't have a serious problem with overeating or body image, but it's been six months since your doctor told you to make some changes in your food choices and you haven't been able to do it to save your life.

Whatever category you belong in, you've probably said, "I guess I just like food too much." Of course you like food. Everybody does. We're supposed to like it so

Some Things Food Addicts May Think

. . . .

- This time will be different
- I ate too much (or gained weight) so I'm a bad person
- No one else eats like I do
- If you really knew me, you wouldn't like me
- I'm fat and disgusting
- I broke my diet so I'm a failure
- Since I ate that cookie, it means I've blown it and have to eat a quart of ice cream
- I've lost weight now so life is supposed to be perfect
- I've lost weight now so I'm cured
- I'll just have a little bit
- I'll get back on my diet tomorrow
- Eating will make me feel better
- I have to eat something to get through this tragedy/term paper/telephone call
- A *venti cappuccino* is really just a big cup of coffee

- When I lose weight, I'll be beautiful
- When I lose weight, my husband/wife/lover will love me (or I'll find a husband/wife/lover who'll love me)
- When I lose weight, my mother/father/other significant person from my past will love and accept me (even if they're dead)
- When I lose weight, I'll do everything I ever wanted to do
- I feel fat (in response to being full, depressed, premenstrual, or constipated, or as a response to rejection, disappointment, or presumed failure)
- If I eat while I read, it won't count (the same goes for food sampled during cooking)
- I deserve a treat (euphemism for extra food), or I deserve to be punished (food can do that, too)
- Eventually, I'll just have the surgery and lose weight that way

much that we eat it as long as we live and live as long as we can. That's nature's way. It's only when food seems to choose us instead of our choosing it that something is wrong. Any time we stuff ourselves, starve ourselves, or eat something we know to be harmful, we're mistreating ourselves in ways that we don't deserve. When we do any of these things repeatedly, we establish a self-destructive and self-defeating pattern. When we want to stop but can't, we're addicted.

Some would argue with that terminology. They would say that food is not universally addictive like heroin or even selectively addictive like alcohol. They might argue that food can cause, at worst, a behavioral dependence. The phenomenon of craving, however, exists in food addiction as in any other kind. It was powerful enough to send me out on foot at midnight in search of caramels. I once had cravings so strong I took leftover cake from an office wastebasket, brushed off the debris, and ate all but the cardboard plate.

I also know that food can be the object of addiction because I see others and myself recovering by using the same principles of transformation that work for other addictions. The only real difference in getting over a food addiction as opposed to an addiction to alcohol is one of abstemiousness versus abstinence. Alcoholics stop drinking alcohol. Drug addicts stop using mood-altering drugs. Food addicts can't give up eating, but we can stop eating for a fix. Recovery is a delicate balance somewhere between the binge and the diet. That's where we abandon the struggle and find sanity and peace of mind.

The dictionary defines recovery as "to get back." For me it has meant getting back some surprising things—the years I lost to binge-eating, for instance. I spent so much of my earlier life in the disease that even though I'm well over fifty, I delight in looking and feeling younger than I am. I'm able to use the nutritional knowledge that I had in abundance (food addicts love learning about food) but could never apply. I've even gotten back the joy of eating. What I did before was drugging, and it was seldom pleasant to my stomach or my conscience. Eating is a pleasure today—that's how it should be. But it's a peripheral pleasure, not the center of my world. And this is not some new, post-diet euphoria: it's been like this for me, one day following another, for nearly twenty-five years.

I once hated the way that I ate but couldn't change it. The difference started when I gave up willpower for the power of love—love for myself and from myself, for others and from them, and grounded in the love that is also power. I'm comfortable calling that God. You can call it whatever you like. It has, by any name, provided an answer where there seemed to be none, and a life beyond the fix that's filled with hope and humor and expectation. Tapping into this power is essential for addicts to live again, and my hunch is that some of that same power is needed for almost anyone to make major lifestyle changes that last. If you do not believe in miracles, or if you think that they don't happen anymore, just come to my house for dinner.

Some Things People Say to Food Addicts
(that don't help at all)

. . . .

- Use a little willpower
- Push yourself away from the table
- I've got this great diet for you
- Just eat less
- How could you let yourself get this way?
- I need to be perfectly honest with you (followed by almost anything)
- You have such a pretty face
- I remember when you wore a size 6 (or 8 or 14)
- Your sister/brother/friend trimmed down so nicely
- I'll come over at six tomorrow morning and we'll go out for a run
- Come on, you have to shape up if you want to attract the ladies (or men)
- I don't know how to tell you this, but do you realize you have a weight problem?
- You look perfectly fine—well, except you could lose a few pounds
- You're too old to change how you eat (or you're too young not to)

- I'm only concerned about your health
- You know, gluttony is a sin
- Take one of these pills whenever you get hungry
- Beauty is only skin deep anyhow
- Do what I did and put a sign on the refrigerator that says "Oink!"
- You can have just one (or, a little won't hurt this once)
- I baked these especially for you
- You'd feel so much better about yourself if you lost a little weight
- I clipped out this article about how much being overweight shortens life expectancy
- I lost five pounds taking these great vitamins—in fact, I'm selling them now
- You just need to get hold of yourself (with or without an addendum about how much of yourself there is to get hold of)

CHAPTER TWO

THE BODY AND THE SPIRIT

Like stepchildren in fairy tales, our bodies get blamed for a lot. When we criticize them, we put ourselves down, too. If you've ever said, "I hate my thighs," or "I used to be pretty but now I'm a wreck," or "Look at this fat—I'm really disgusting," you were playing the role of your own evil stepmother.

Your weight may be a problem, but it isn't *the* problem. It's a symptom—almost always a symptom of an unhealthy or unloving relationship with food. You can be rid of the symptom while the real problem flourishes. Getting thin is not a cure. Any size 2 woman with bulimia can attest to that. Nevertheless, if you deal with the cause of the overweight, your body will reflect wellness, balance, and beauty that go far beyond how you look in something clingy.

There's a cause-and-effect chain with which you need to be familiar:

INNER MALAISE leads to DESTRUCTIVE EATING
which (usually) leads to OVERWEIGHT.

The components of *inner malaise* are fear and discontent, stress and impaired self-image, emotional leftovers from childhood, or anything else that stands between us and a reasonable degree of contentment.

Instead of starting at the source, though, we've traditionally gone after the obvious, the weight. And why not? We can see it. We can even weigh it, for heaven's sake. But when it's gone (via diet, exercise, liposuction, even gastric bypass), the inner malaise can still be active, resulting in further destructive eating. In fact, as long as the inner malaise goes unchecked, even dieting is destructive eating (or destructive non-eating). It will eventually lead to gaining back the lost weight, or to some variation on the theme, such as bulimia or exercise addiction.

This is not to say that there are no physiological reasons why some people struggle more than others with overweight. Scientists have found evidence that low levels of a hormone called leptin may cause some men and women—perhaps ten percent of heavy people—to store extra fat. There's also a gene called lipoprotein lipase (LPL) that determines whether a particular body is better at using calories consumed or storing them as fat. (Even these genetic factors can be offset to some degree with exercise and the low-fat, plant-based eating program we'll discuss in the second half of this book.)

For some people with food and weight problems, refined sugars and greasy, salty snacks seem to cause an addictive reaction that leads to overeating. Too much fat in your diet can result in too much fat on your body, and lack of exercise can lower your metabolic rate, encouraging fat storage. Dieting itself is also a factor. The deprivation of dieting can cause a physical and emotional backlash that Neal Barnard, MD, has called *restrained eater phenomenon.* "The body cannot distinguish dieting from starvation," Dr. Barnard writes in his book *The Power of Your Plate.* "We are automatically driven to gorge ourselves in anticipation of recurrent famine."

Another problem with dieting is that it usually limits the range of tastes we're permitted to enjoy. According to the time-honored healing system of Ayurveda, we need to experience the full spectrum of tastes in order to feel satisfied. The typical Westerner eats foods that are primarily sweet and salty, largely depriving the taste buds of sour, bitter, pungent (spicy), and astringent sensations. (*Astringent* refers to the clean and slightly dry taste of foods such as beans, apples, potatoes, and cabbage.) Dieters restrict themselves even further. When we don't get all six tastes each day, preferably at every lunch and dinner, we can feel that something is missing. We think that we need second helpings or dessert or cafeteria-style evenings of one snack after another. One solution to taste deprivation is to include a bit of the Indian condiment chutney, made from a variety of fruits and spices, with every meal.

Another is to eat adequately from a wide variety of "real foods" and not live in mortal terror of their calorie content.

Knowing about the various physical reasons that may underlie an off-kilter relationship with food is different from *doing* something about them. What is it that keeps so many people from doing what they know would bring them what they want? For a great many people—and only you can decide if you're one of them—inner malaise blocks their attempts to put into practice the good things they already know about nutrition and a healthy lifestyle.

Some people have realized that attacking the weight is a hopeless maneuver, and they have proposed alternative plans of action that focus on the second part of the equation: the eating itself. Their strategy is generally behavior modification—techniques such as taking small bites and putting the fork down between them, or forgoing the fork altogether and giving chopsticks a try, or perhaps not eating alone or not eating after seven PM. These can be positive practices, but most of the time they fail over the long haul. Why? Because our actions ultimately grow out of ourselves. Unless we change, our actions aren't likely to change in any long-term way.

On the other hand, when the inner malaise itself is addressed, both harmful eating patterns and the fat storage that follows lose their source and sustenance. Tiny miracles transpire one by one. We take those smaller bites. We aren't hanging onto the fork as if it were our firstborn babe. Breathing gets easier. Clothes get looser. And although we never asked for this one, life gets better. It has to, because it's being lived in a new and decidedly better way.

Healing at the Desire Level

When healing comes like this, from within, it's healing at the desire level. It's no longer wanting a candy bar and settling for an orange; it's wanting an orange—organic, juicy, in season—and relishing every bite of it. This doesn't mean that there will never again be food choices to make. There are healthful and unhealthful food choices just as there are healthful and unhealthful life choices. Only by dealing with the inner malaise, though, are we able to truly make choices about what we eat. Otherwise, the choices are made for us and we usually regret them.

Phase Out Fat Days

. . . .

Do you ever have fat days? On fat days you feel fat regardless of your Body Mass Index or the size of your jeans. These days can be precipitated by eating way too much, a little too much, or just what you think is too much. They can also be brought on by such seeming irrelevancies as having dirty hair or an argument with your mother. Losing weight isn't a fully satisfactory response to fat days since they're so subjective. For people with anorexia, every day is a fat day, even if they're near death from lack of nourishment.

The rest of us may laugh off fat days, but they're not laughable, because they're days when you love yourself less than you deserve. You're lovable every day. You can't force yourself to believe that, but you can allow the possibility that it's true to enter your world view. Allowing for such possibilities is a spiritual activity because it takes place deep within you.

A young woman once said to me, "When I'm 150 and the scale is going up, I'm the fattest, ugliest person on Earth, but when I'm 150 and the scale is coming down, I'm absolutely beautiful." Perhaps you relate. This woman has long since recovered from compulsive eating and the feeling of "going up" and "coming down" affects her today only on airplanes and elevators.

Spiritual recovery means more than an end to eating for a fix. It also implies befriending your body. You don't wait to do that until after you've reached some arbitrary goal weight. You do it today, the first day that you put your food choices in the hands of a loving Higher Power.

The imaging ability of your mind that can be twisted to give you fat days can be uplifted to give you attractive and healthy days. As these days accrue, your physical body will catch up with your mental image. Since the body is subject to physical laws, it will take some time for its form to change, but the time it takes for you to be happy and to have an attractive, healthy day is no time at all.

When we turn to unhealthful or excessive food (or any other damaging substance or practice) in order to feel better, it's because something is missing in our lives. Although it seems that what we lack is outside ourselves—the right job, the right mate, the right body, the right memories—the emptiness is core-deep. To make satisfying, lasting changes in how we nourish our bodies, we must learn to get some vital nourishment from within. We do that by connecting with our spiritual selves—by making practical contact with a Higher Power, whatever we perceive that to be.

If you can get past the binge/diet syndrome by some other means, terrific. I couldn't. I'd stressed my resolve and my willpower until, like overworked peasants, they revolted. That insidious urge to smooth life's rough edges with a nibble that could turn into a nightmare would overtake me just when I was convinced I had everything under control. My intelligence and good intentions were of no more use than lighting fixtures in a house with no wiring. I needed power and I didn't have it. I was desperate to tap into a Higher Power, one that would always be there.

It was such a strange notion. My problem seemed so physical. I ate quantities of physical food and it showed quantitatively on my physical body, yet paradoxically the answer to my problem was spiritual. It didn't make sense to me at first and it may not make sense to you until you realize that, as human beings, we are like icebergs. Our physical selves are only the tip of our totality. There's so much more beneath the surface. We're splendid beings with complex emotions and intellects, and underlying our hearts, minds, and bodies is a spiritual essence. It's uniquely ours, yet it connects us to every living thing. It connects us to life itself.

The part of you that shows—your body—is important because it's a part of you and you are important. You can think of your body as the vehicle in which you journey through this life; or as your radio receiver picking up signals from the outside world; or an instrument in an orchestra, allowing you to play your music for the rest of us. A symphony needs French horns and oboes; cellos and violins; tiny, tinkling triangles and booming timpani. In the same way, there's a place for each one of us.

Abusing food can interfere with your ability to appreciate your special physical self. In an all-out binge, you have to cut off diplomatic relations between the body and the mind. Since it's a rare person who consciously wants to be miserable, most people who binge separate their conscious (thinking) selves from their sensory (physical) selves by reading, surfing the web, driving, or watching TV while they eat. They absentmindedly grab snacks throughout the day or sneak tastes while preparing a meal. Swearing off the distractions that remove you from the present moment may seem like the antidote, but it isn't. If you have the need to binge, you'll find a way to shut off your mind, with all its *shoulds* and *oughts* and *know betters*—and go for the food.

The need to binge is a spiritual hunger. It can only be assuaged with spiritual food. The soul lives on love the way a koala bear lives on eucalyptus leaves. All genuine love is good—love from family, your friends, your dog or cat—but the kind that you need for this purpose can't be filtered through anyone else. It has to come from the source: love that's within you so you don't have to look for it, that's already yours so you don't have to earn it, that can't stop loving you so you don't have to worry about losing it. Once you realize that this love exists and that it's available to you with no questions asked, you'll be eager to put into practice the principles that you'll learn in this book. You begin by:

(1) Accepting that your food problem is serious, that you can't deal with it on your own
(2) Opening your mind to the idea that a Higher Power can change things
(3) Allowing that Higher Power—call it love, call it God, call it whatever feels right to you—to work some wonders in your life.

If you're familiar with the Twelve Steps of Alcoholics Anonymous (adopted by Overeaters Anonymous, Gamblers Anonymous, Debtors Anonymous, and numerous other groups), you'll recognize these three concepts as an interpretation of the first three steps. People in the anonymous programs sometimes abbreviate them as: "(1) I can't. (2) God can. (3) I'll let Him (or Her or It)." However worded, this formula is common to men and women of all ages and cultures who have built or rebuilt their lives on a spiritual basis, letting go of old ways that didn't work and inviting in something new that does.

A Lifetime Adventure

Spiritualizing your thoughts and attitudes is an adventure that can last a lifetime. To instigate the process, particularly as it affects your eating, take the following actions today and every day for the next month:

- Each morning before your feet touch the floor, ask your Higher Power to help you eat reasonably that day. At night say "Thank you," even if your eating (or your day) wasn't perfect.
- When you're at the mirror to put on your makeup or shave, look yourself in the eye and say, "I love you just the way you are." You don't have to believe it yet. Just do it.
- Read over the "Revolutionary Concepts" (page 17) every morning and evening.
- Spend some quiet time by yourself every single day—at least ten minutes' worth. If you have to take this time in the bathtub to get privacy, fine. During this period, read over the first three of the Twelve Steps in their original form (see Appendix), change the word "alcohol" in Step 1 to "food," and think about these steps. Do you really believe that you're powerless over your addiction or is there something else you'd like to try? Can you contemplate the possibility that a Higher Power could help? Can you consider making a decision to put that Higher Power in charge of your will and your life? (Writing your thoughts on this in a journal isn't required, but it can be helpful.)
- Do not diet. Think instead in terms of refraining from eating for a fix one day at a time. Enjoy three reasonable meals each day. (If you have a health problem that calls for eating more often, do what your doctor tells you. If there's no medical reason for you to eat more than three times a day, eat breakfast, lunch, and dinner, period, no excuses.) Before each meal ask your Higher Power to help you eat wisely. If you want to eat at other times, converse with your Higher Power. If a meal is delayed or if for some other reason you are genuinely, physically hungry, have a piece of fruit. Eat it slowly. Enjoy it. Then get back to living.
- Do at least two nice things for yourself today—one nice thing that you think you should do (make the bed, floss your teeth, swim laps) and one that's just for fun (take a bubble bath, go to a movie, have coffee with a friend).
- Enlist some support. At the very least, read this book with another person and help each other along. You'll do yourself a great favor, however, if you connect with a support group already organized that uses proven principles to help food addicts recover. OA—www.overeatersanonymous.org. This group will

teach you how to incorporate the Twelve Steps into your life while providing an unparalleled support system of people who understand the disease of compulsive eating and how to recover from it. There's no charge to be a member, and there are OA meetings in cities and towns across America and around the world, as well as telephone and online meetings. OA is a recovery program, not a diet club.

If you're feeling overwhelmed by all this, take a deep breath, blow it out, and let yourself relax. It's a lot to process. Give yourself time to let these notions settle. You may want to read this chapter more than once before you go further. You're embarking on a transformational journey. That's no small thing and some trepidation is normal. Old patterns are going to be replaced and they don't want to get fired.

While you're making layoffs, you may also want to consider trading any old images of a punishing, wrathful deity for one that loves you no matter what. Or maybe you need to revamp your concept of a Higher Power that may be nice enough, but that seems too mythical for your rational self to buy into a concept that makes sense to you today. The idea is to develop your own understanding of a Higher Power that isn't just interested in great, cosmic events but one that's within you and is therefore interested in you and seeing you out of your food addiction. Start with whatever image works for you and allow it to change over time if you need to. Just get used to being loved unconditionally, weird as that might seem if you've never felt it before.

Coming up with your own concept doesn't mean that you're "inventing God." It means that you're accepting the idea that there's more to life than what we see, and using your gift of creative thought to come up with an understanding of what is beyond understanding. Einstein said, "I want to know God's thoughts. The rest are details." He didn't say, "Because I am a really smart genius, I know God's thoughts," only that he *wanted* to. If Einstein was allowed to seek and explore and extrapolate in the realm of the unknown, so are you.

Whether you realize it or not, you, like Einstein, are spiritual. Do not think for an instant because the solution to food addiction is spiritual that food addicts themselves are somehow lacking in spiritual potential. True, in the midst of a binge anyone's spirituality is on temporary hold, but your inherent spiritual identity persists. It doesn't go anywhere just because you're carrying too much weight or you are in some other way misaligned in the eating/exercise/body image area.

Revolutionary Concepts

. . . .

These revolutionary concepts aren't for overthrowing governments, they're the beginner's basics for revolutionizing your relationship with your body and how you feed it. Read them over every morning and evening for the next month, paying particular attention to those with which you may feel uncomfortable. It's possible that those don't apply to you, but it's more likely that they're precisely the ones that can mean the most in your recovery.

- You're acceptable right now, regardless of what you ate yesterday or what the scale has to say about you

- Abusing food is a sign of internal imbalance, and overcoming it is largely an inside job

- Food addiction is serious and, like other addictions, progressive. Few genuine addicts have ever recovered without undergoing an inner metamorphosis

- Your spirituality is personal. You don't have to take on someone else's brand

- You're a spiritual being living in a physical body. Your body is an integral part of the totality that is you

- Your body is not an independent entity. Instead, it reflects what's going on inside you emotionally, mentally, and spiritually

- It's OK to feel beautiful right now. If you wait until you're thin to feel beautiful, you may never get there

- If you don't eat for a fix today, that long string of tomorrows that seems so foreboding will take care of itself

- Your body is not your enemy. You and your body are in this together

- Having a food addiction doesn't make you a bad person or even a weak one. Both medicine and psychology recognize addiction as an illness, not a moral issue

- You don't have to be perfect to get well, and it's even OK to be a little bit scared

- Ideas that you're not sure of can be tried out, like taking a car on a test drive. If, for example, the thought of a spiritual solution to your food problem doesn't seem logical, you can consider it as a possibility and test it out as a hypothesis.

All the inner growth you've done up to this point counts, too. Only you and your Higher Power know how far you've had to come to get here, to the point where you can honestly look at yourself and what you're eating. Give yourself credit for getting here and resist the urge to compare yourself to anyone else. All that matters now is that you've suffered with this long enough. It's your turn to be free—body and spirit.

CHAPTER THREE

GETTING TO POINT ZERO

A race is only fair when everybody starts at the starting line. If life were a race, though, some of us would have a to run a veritable marathon just to get to that starting point at which everyone else seems fresh and rested, eager to take off. I call that place Point Zero. At Point Zero, you're unencumbered and your chances for winning are as good as anybody's. Eating for a fix, however, can keep you from getting there.

Healthy people meet every new day, every new dilemma, every new project from the level ground of Point Zero. Because they like themselves, they're comfortable with life and aren't likely to become addicted to anything. They're not perfect and they don't need to be. They are, however, at home in their own skins and in the world around them. When they have difficulties, they're able to get the help they need and use the help they get, whether it comes from family, friends, professionals, or their own inner resources. They rebound well from adversity and although they may lose many things in life, hope isn't one of them. At Point Zero, there's always hope, spirited challenge, and limitless potential.

Addictive behavior keeps Point Zero elusive. Food addicts now in recovery have described it in the following ways:

"I felt like I was in an invisible box and couldn't get out. People kept offering me advice and ideas that I couldn't use because I couldn't get out of the box to try them. I see now that I'd built the box myself and I'd built it with a tight-fitting lid."

"There was one awful thing in my life: the way I ate. I was really angry that I couldn't do anything about it since I seemed to be so good at everything else. It seemed like a terrible blight to me, a stigma."

"My life looked OK. I had a lot going on and was busy all the time. But when I was alone, something always seemed to be missing. I was experiencing a quiet desperation. I acted happy, you know, 'jolly,' but I was so sad."

As you can see from the diagram on page 36, Point Zero is a sort of alchemical crossroads at which the old baggage of sub-zero attitudes and actions turns into golden qualities. Obsessive eating no longer fits. You accept life on its own terms. You're a participant in it instead of a spectator. You see fear transmuted into safe, healing, unconditional love. It provides the foundation for the best possible relationships with yourself, other people, and the myriad things that make up your life: your work, your interests, your finances and, of course, your food.

When you clear away what stands between you and Point Zero, you'll be able to tap into that love, which has always been available, more easily than ever before. Once you do, you'll find yourself showing up when life is passing the good stuff your way, and when circumstances aren't the best, you won't be brought down so far with them.

The fear-motivated thought-and-action patterns you see on the diagram beneath Point Zero lead away from self-love and self-care. It doesn't make you a bad person to be acquainted with those patterns, they are simply thoughts and actions that don't work to bring you what you want in life. They worked at one time or you wouldn't have developed them. They were powerful mechanisms that were once useful but now do more harm than good, like an old pair of glasses that used to help you see better but now make everything a blur.

Using food or extra weight as a buffer between yourself and life is one way to keep old patterns intact and stay negative, in the red, below Point Zero. This does not mean that because you and I have histories of misusing food we are, or ever were, less valuable than the next person. The fact that we're alive makes us remarkable. Besides, you can come from a respected family, be highly intelligent, well-educated, and gainfully employed but still feel sub-zero inside.

It may manifest as feeling out of place much of the time or as if you're some-how different from other people. You may be tired of trying to reach some invisi-ble goal or meet some impossible standard. You may recognize as your own some of the sub-zero thinking patterns in "A Mental Makeover" later in this chapter. However much or little you relate to these examples, if you're still using food in a way that you're uncomfortable with (or if you're not right now but you're afraid you will again), there's some distance between you and the freedom you'll find at Point Zero.

Your mission, then, is to get to Point Zero from wherever you're starting. In one sense, there isn't far to go—only about twelve inches, the distance from your head to your heart. In terms of consciousness, however, this may be the most mean-ingful journey you've ever taken. You won't make it to Point Zero alone or by sheer effort or willpower. You need to resign yourself to being the passenger on this trip: Love (God, Higher Power) will do the driving. You only need to get in the car. Your willingness to do this employs your will to the best advantage.

You started on the trek to Point Zero in the preceding chapter when you came to grips with the fact that you can't handle your food problem by yourself, when you allowed yourself to believe that a Higher Power could make the difference, and you decided to let that loving Power be in charge of things. You'll reach Point Zero as you clean up the past and learn to live fearlessly and productively in the present. There are five things that you must do:

- Become more honest than you've ever been
- Postpone eating for a fix
- Sit with your feelings
- Make peace with the past and with other people
- Expand your comfort zone

Underlying all these admonitions are spiritual verities that have, over time, shown themselves to make people's lives better. Because truth is well told in fable, I will introduce each of the five ways for getting to Point Zero with a story.

Become More Honest

There was once a shaman whose fame for miraculous healings spread far and wide. The people of his country were astounded by the miracles he performed and discoursed among themselves about how he accomplished them. "He becomes as tiny as a gnat," one suggested, "and goes into the sick body, sees what is wrong, and eats it away."

"No," argued another. "He becomes as tall as the sky and lifts the sick person up to the gods. It is they who do the magic."

The shaman overheard this conversation and gently interrupted: "I am no larger or smaller than either of you, my friends. And the healings that you see are not magic. I have simply spoken the truth in earnestness for such a long time that my words cannot be false. When I say that someone is well, he can be nothing else."

Honesty is not optional if you want to live without a food problem. In *The Answer to Addiction*, John Burns and three other recovered alcoholics explain it this way: "You connect to God by means of the truth. And you connect with the truth by stopping lying."

Most of us don't think of ourselves as liars, but a solid commitment to honesty is such a rarity that borderline dishonesty passes as acceptable and is even commendable. It's usually little things. A waiter forgets to charge for the appetizer and the customer ignores it, or a six-year-old is passed off as five to get free admission to the theme park or a free ride on the bus. The individual incidents don't amount to much, but they reflect a pervasive lack of regard for honesty in general. It wasn't long ago that "I give you my word" was as good as collateral, but that's no longer the case. The result is that it takes a lot for people to trust one another. Even worse: we're often not sure we can trust ourselves.

Addiction breeds dishonesty, usually in subtle ways. "I really didn't eat much dinner" (but you finished off all the leftovers). "I just didn't like anything I tried on" (nothing fit). "I think I'll stay in tonight and get some work done" (being home alone is a great way to binge in peace).

To become more honest, even if you believe you're already as honest as you need to be, *The Answer to Addiction* offers the following suggestions: "As a starter, stop lying to yourself about your addicted condition. . . . Next, stop lying to get out of jams or to smooth off the rough edges of life. Don't lie for the sake of peace; don't lie when common sense invites you to do so; don't lie to cover up your past; don't lie on job applications, expense accounts, or tax returns; don't lie to your boss; don't lie to your husband or wife. Just don't lie. When you fail in this resolve (as you will), admit it promptly. And don't indulge failure—that is, don't fail any more than you have to."

An excellent place to initiate a commitment to honesty—although probably the most frightening—is with your eating. First, be honest with yourself about what you're putting into your mouth. Just because you eat something quickly and get rid of the wrapper, or because there isn't anyone else around, doesn't mean you didn't eat it. Did you really have "a few chips" or was it a bag? If it was a bag, acknowledge that it was indeed a bag. Denying reality doesn't change reality. Dishonesty, however, brings on dangerous rationalization: "I just had a few, so it won't make any difference if I have a few more."

While you're at it, it won't hurt to be honest about your weight. In a lot of ways, weight is a silly measurement of anything. It can fluctuate from day to day, and scales vary in their readings. Adding some weight, when it's muscle, actually makes you leaner. But let's face it: you know just about how much you weigh. Tell the truth about it, especially to yourself.

Being truthful will hasten your progress toward freedom from the food fix more assuredly than any other single action. When your personal code of ethics includes both accepting the truth and speaking the truth, you'll see remarkable improvements in your life. Commit yourself to a totally honest day and see how much easier that makes it to eat reasonably. You'll also go to sleep that night with a particularly peaceful feeling.

Having people around you that you can trust with honest confidences will assist you in your experiment with expanded honesty. These may be the people closest to you, although sometimes being upfront with those very significant others is tougher than with people more peripherally connected to you. Connecting with other food addicts who are committed to recovery, like those you'll come to know if you affiliate with Overeaters Anonymous, can be a real blessing in this regard. If

Honesty Exercises

. . . .

- Drive within the speed limit, even when you're sure that you wouldn't get caught if you didn't.

- When you hear yourself putting yourself down verbally or mentally ("I'm a slob," "I can't do anything right"), delete that thought. Blanket put-downs of yourself or others do not reflect the truth.

- When you're wrong, say so.

- If a certain food has always been a problem for you ("One bite is too many and a thousand aren't enough"), face the fact and leave that food alone.

- Abandon the cover-up, for yourself or others. If you forget to return a call, say "I forgot." If your child didn't do her homework, don't help out with a subterfuge.

- Share with someone else exactly what you're eating, or at least write down honestly what you're eating and share it with yourself.

- Shop for food honestly. Do you really need to serve the scout troop your favorite kind of cookie? Are you truly expecting someone who dearly loves caramels to "just drop by"?

- Be completely honest about your life and your feelings with one or more people whom you trust.

- Eat the same way when you're alone as when you're with people and vice versa.

- Be who you are wherever you are. If you have a chameleon suit, trade it in. Your beliefs, opinions, and preferences needn't be altered to fit one group or occasion and then another.

- When you find yourself exaggerating, bring the story down to size.

- Remember the important truth for food addicts: Alone, our prospects are grim, but there's a spiritual solution. Act on that truth.

nothing else, be sure there's one other person in this world with whom you're willing to be absolutely honest, and share with him or her on a regular basis.

In time, dishonesty simply won't feel comfortable any longer. This doesn't mean you'll become harsh toward other people. "Honest to a fault" can describe those who like to criticize. With honesty based on love, however, you'll be able to speak kindly and truthfully. You'll also know when it's best to say nothing at all. This sort of intuition comes about as a result of your commitment to the truth. As that commitment grows, your true self—the one that's at Point Zero, healthy, happy, and addiction-free—will start to emerge.

Postpone Eating for a Fix

A severe storm destroyed all the huts in a small village. In the days that followed, the villagers were hard at work reconstructing their dwellings before the next rain. One man, however, sat at the site where his hut had been, gathering no building materials and lifting no tools. "Why are you not building a shelter?" his neighbors queried. "The rains will come again soon."

The man was unmoved. "God took my house from me. He owes me another. I am waiting for God to build it." It was not long before the rains again poured down upon the village. The homeless man beat on the doors of his neighbors' houses, but the neighbors thought him lazy and would not let him in. He disappeared into the forest.

Some believe that he perished, but the wise tell their children how the man lost his senses in the woodland and lives there yet, wild and half-starved, his home the branches of a tree. "That," they warn the children, "is the best house you can expect if you refuse to give God a helping hand."

You can offer that helping hand with your willingness to postpone the fix. When love motivates your life, it will motivate your eating. A healthy relationship with food is one of the gifts that love—genuine love for yourself as well as for others—will bring into your life. You accept this gift every time you refrain from using food for the wrong reasons.

It may seem paradoxical to suggest that you do so since the first step in recovery is the admission that you can't control your eating. That surrender, however, implies a transfer of power: You trade personal power for Love's power, God's power. Therefore, even if you think that you cannot possibly do it, you'll be able to postpone eating for a fix. Recovering addicts of all stripes use the "twenty-four-hours-at-a-time" method, which means that you only have to worry about not eating for a fix one day at a time. Deal with the twenty-four-hour period you're living through right now, not the one tomorrow or a month from now. In dealing with other compulsions, it means not popping the first pill, or placing the first bet, or lighting the first cigarette. In this case it's not swallowing the first inappropriate mouthful.

We're not able to say, "Starting this Monday, I'm going on 1,200 calories until I've lost twenty-five pounds." We've done that and sooner or later it always backfired. What we are able to do is refrain from inappropriate eating today, just this day, from the time we awaken in the morning until we go to sleep at night. Neither yesterday nor tomorrow has any place in practicing a new way of life. It can only be done in the immediacy of the present.

As you work with spiritual ideas, your impulses to use food in unhealthy ways will diminish. Eventually, only in rare incidences will the urge to turn to food surface. When it does, you'll actually appreciate it as a signal that something isn't right inside. By then you'll have ample tools to use to get for yourself what you really need at that moment—probably some emotional or spiritual sustenance that can't be stored in a refrigerator. A supportive community, such as Overeaters Anonymous or something like it, can be invaluable at these times as well.

With your growing inner strength and the help of others, you can learn what you need from the feelings you're experiencing, long before they lead you to the kitchen or the deli. In the beginning, however, you may have the desire to eat inappropriately rather often. Inappropriate eating includes situations like these:

- It's eleven AM. You're at the office. Your boss has told you to redo a report you've worked on all week. Lunch isn't for another hour, but as you look around, you think that you could eat this morning's mail, a telephone, and a couple of laptops.
- You're in bed with a cold. You just had a substantial lunch but it didn't taste like anything. Besides, there's nobody around to take care of you. A little something would really help, you know, a little sweet thing or a little salty thing.
- You've stopped smoking, but you miss the pleasant prolonging of dinner that a cigarette used to provide. Lately you've substituted extra helpings and second desserts.

- There's no avoiding it: This is cleaning day. You had breakfast and you've descended on the bathrooms. You're fine on the basins and tubs, but then come the floors. You hate doing floors. This seems like an ideal time for a snack.
- Your son's music lesson lasts an hour. It's not mealtime and you're not really hungry, but the only pleasant thing to do between dropping him off and picking him up is to go somewhere for a bite.
- Your spouse brought home some cookies yesterday. They're the good ones. You know in your heart of hearts that eating one means eating the package, but you eat one (and then the package) anyway.
- It's the middle of the night. You're up raiding the refrigerator and may not even remember how you got there. (Night eating can be a serious problem and professional help may be a valuable adjunct in the recovery process. Nevertheless, proven spiritual principles in tandem with group support have relieved all sorts of problem eaters, even the after-hours variety.)

Remember that as love-powered living becomes a habit, trying situations can present themselves and you'll much less often have the urge to respond to them with eating. When it does crop up, the technique of postponement will prove invaluable. Start with a twenty-four-hour solution. This is the day you're concerned about. You may need to shorten the time frame and be willing to put off the fix for two hours or one hour or for fifteen minutes.

And what good does that do? Plenty. For one thing, if you've just finished a meal and want more, it may simply reflect physiological lag time. It takes about 20 minutes for the satiation center in your brain to register that you're full. When you allow that period of time to elapse, your desire to continue eating may abate and you won't need to do anything else. In addition, you can use that postponement time to get yourself centered. This is particularly important if you want to eat for emotional rather than physical reasons, even if you can't at the time tell one from the other.

Centering means finding that point of peace within yourself. It's there. It's there now, even if you're holding this book in your right hand and a doughnut in your left. The point of peace is with you when you're feeling angry, anxious, scared, or tired—and you can find it. Once there, you can more easily connect with the power of love that will do for you what food never could.

There are a variety of calming techniques such as relaxation and meditation to bring you to this state of mind (see Chapter Four, "Looking In, Reaching Out"). Prayer or meditation at the time you want to open the refrigerator door can be of real help, provided that you truly want the help. "Preventive prayer" or making a routine of daily quiet time can fill empty places in advance so that you won't look to whatever is in the fridge to do it.

In addition to meditation and prayer, you can go from frantic to stable by engaging in any nondestructive activity that you enjoy. It's a smart move to make a list of the feel-good things you like to do, because if you wait until you want to eat everything that can't run faster than you, the only feel-good thing you'll be able to remember is eating. Keep your list in your computer (ideally on the desktop where you'll see it) and make hard copies for your bedside table, your desk at home and at the office, your car, and of course somewhere in the kitchen. Your list will be your own. I call mine *Happy Stuff* and it looks like this:

- Meeting my daughter at Starbucks
- Organizing some small space in my life, maybe a drawer or a closet
- Comedy, even on TV
- Communing with my cat
- Hot baths
- Seeing a movie (extra points if it's a documentary)
- Going to the gym (technically, *leaving* the gym is the happy part, but I don't get that without showing up)
- Delicious music, especially show tunes
- Stimulating conversation with someone whose company delights me
- Walking in New York City
- A date with my handsome husband

My full list is even longer. Happiness lists tend to grow as your awareness of the many delicious things in life broadens. Obviously, the desire to eat inappropriately can strike when you aren't free to hop in the bathtub or stroll in Central Park. Then you need immediate postponement techniques that also connect you with your spiritual source. Here are some examples:

- Read a paragraph or two of something helpful
- Call someone you know to be supportive of your desire to eat rationally
- Change your environment, even for a few minutes, like using your coffee break to get outside, walk around a little, breathe some fresher air
- Write down how you're feeling and you may be surprised by what comes out; putting emotions and confusions down in black and white can be both revealing and freeing (you may think of it as praying on paper)
- Get by yourself, even it it's in the washroom, for a brief quiet time
- Ask your Higher Power to help you get through the craving until it passes.

There's no such thing as a craving that doesn't wear itself out. Most people never realize that. They either give in to the craving as soon as it surfaces or fight it and end up exhausted. They can't see that cravings exit if they're denied attention. Another effective postponement technique is also significant in getting to Point Zero. That is learning to sit with your feelings.

Sit with Your Feelings

Long ago there lived a woman who believed that her house was possessed by demons. She called on the local priest to exorcise them. The priest performed the proper rites, but within a week the woman was again at the rectory gate. "My house is once more possessed," she cried. The priest performed the ritual a second time and instructed his parishioner to return home.

Not a day had passed before the woman beseeched him a third time to cleanse her house. This request the good father refused. "The terrors that alarm you," he told her, "are less within the walls of your house than within those of your mind. You must confront these spirits yourself."

"But won't you give me something to help, a vial of holy water or a sacred crucifix?" the woman pleaded.

"I will give you something," the priest replied. "I will give you a holy stool." He took from the corner a simple wooden hassock. It didn't look particularly holy, but the woman took it nonetheless. When she entered her house, demons abounded from cellar to loft.

"I am lost," she thought. "Even with this holy stool as a weapon, I could never fight them all." She sat on the stool to await her fate, but the instant she was comfortably seated, the demons disappeared. The woman was convinced from that day forward that the cleric's gift indeed bore divine power. The priest, however, knew that the demons departed simply because she had been willing to sit with them. And he missed his favorite footstool for the rest of his life.

For all our contemporary sophistication, many of us are terrified by demons. The ones we fear aren't supernatural, they're our own feelings. We label some as negative—grief, remorse, anger, wounded pride—and feel justified in avoiding contact with them. Sometimes, however, we're equally uncomfortable with positive emotions. We're cautious about accepting compliments (we may not deserve them), feeling too good (we might jinx it), or even loving someone (they could go away). A tried-and-true way to keep from feeling anything is to overeat. You've heard the phrase "to stuff your face." It could just as easily be stated "to stuff your feelings."

The surest road for getting past anything difficult or emotional is the one that leads you through without turning to food. In other words, sit with your feelings. The feelings may have to do with a major life upheaval. Sit with them. More likely, the feelings you'd prefer to eat into oblivion result from everyday annoyances, nuisance situations, and solvable problems that will work out whether you choose solution A or solution B. Whether you're meeting tragedy or trivia, you can sit with your feelings without food in your mouth. Each time you do this, the intensity of your desire to abuse food will soften and you will, perhaps without even knowing it, be inviting precious serenity into your world.

What it means to sit with your feelings is simply that: to be with them, feel them, and come to know that they're not demonic forces but rather healers in their own right. Grief is a perfect example. Feeling grief, although certainly not enjoyable, is our part in the necessary process of recovering from a loss. Episodes of grief are precisely timed as if the body and mind share a well-set clock. You cannot grieve too much at once. There's some grieving now, some later. Eventually, when the process has been allowed to complete itself, there's no further need for it.

Other emotions operate similarly. Anger fades. So does elation. They come to pass, not to stay. Every emotion has a purpose and a duration. To get in touch with these, understand them, act on them when appropriate, and then let them go, it's necessary to be present to them. You can't do that while eating a hero sandwich, checking e-mail, and watching the evening news. You do it by releasing the need for *doing* altogether and allowing yourself to simply *be*.

In our society-wide hastiness, it's easy to misinterpret feelings. What feels like hunger may be anger, shame, or fear. These feelings can manifest as a cold, empty sensation in the pit of your stomach. It's no wonder you can confuse this with the need for food. Lots of feelings are similarly lost in translation. What seems like anger toward one person, for instance, may turn out to be anger toward someone else or toward yourself. In sitting with your feelings, you pay attention to them, the way a wise parent knows how to pay attention to an unruly child, to learn what's behind the behavior.

Ideally, giving this sort of attention to feelings means taking some time to sit quietly and purposefully with whatever is going on inside you. This is a skill that will take some practice. You begin by not eating for the time being and doing instead something with less potential for avoiding your feelings. Talking with an understanding person can be a godsend, as can writing in a journal, taking a walk, working in your garden, or booking a massage or some other sort of calming bodywork. Eventually, you'll be able to sit, on a borrowed footstool maybe, with whatever is happening in and around you, and you won't be afraid. As you open yourself to what you feel, you'll find that you become open to what you need. It may be a life coach or a day off or more fresh fruits and vegetables in your diet. As you become aware of these things, it's your job to see that you get what you need.

I can remember when the prospect of voluntarily feeling what I was feeling without deadening it with food seemed about as likely as paying off the national debt from my Christmas savings. With enough reassurance from people who had done it, though, and with bits of practice whenever I could get it, I came to welcome opportunities to be present to my own interior life. It isn't always easy, but when you know that the only dependable way out of uncomfortable feelings is moving through them, the process gets easier. Fears decrease and boredom disappears. Problems cease being crosses to bear and become bridges to cross. And you'll come to expect something wonderful on the other side.

Make Peace with the Past

A Zen story has it that two Buddhist monks were traveling on foot from their monastery to another in a neighboring town. To keep their vow of silence between sunrise and sunset, they walked wordlessly, reverently. After a few hours, they came to a flooded crossing. A finely dressed young woman was attempting to get to the other side, but there seemed no way for her to do this without soiling her garments in the mud. Seeing her plight, one of the monks wordlessly approached and, lifting her carefully, carried her across the rivulet and set her down on the other side. He then continued his silent journey.

When darkness fell, the second monk admonished him. "I am shocked that, given our vows of purity, you blatantly touched a woman today."

"It is true," the first monk replied, "that I carried her in my arms over the water. But you, my brother, have carried her in your mind all day."

We've already talked about living in the present. We don't take the first bite of a binge today. We sit with our feelings in this situation. To place ourselves firmly in the present, however, requires that we be at peace with the past. We cannot move gracefully through a current experience while lugging burdens of judgment, disappointment, guilt, and resentment, many of them from a long time ago. Like the accusing monk in the story, though, we can carry these burdens all day, and sometimes for all our lives.

To deal sanely and compassionately with the past and with all the people in our lives, half of the anonymous programs' Twelve Steps are devoted to personal inventory and personal peacemaking. Reread steps 4 through 9 in The Twelve Steps in Appendix A. You'll see that they begin with a thorough stocktaking (making "a searching and fearless moral inventory") and sharing what's discovered with oneself, another person, and a Higher Power.

It's important not to skip over this because you've done something similar before. Taking an inventory is not an excuse for putting yourself down or blaming yourself for every woe in the world. In fact, a tendency toward excessive self-blame may come out in an inventory as something you wish to be free of. The inventory is not "confession" in the way you may know that term because you won't be looking for rules you've broken. Instead, you'll find the actions and inactions that you're uncomfortable with, that you wish you could change, and that have led (or could lead) to unnecessary food.

The inventory is also not about the buried psychological paraphernalia you might discover in psychotherapy. Surely insights will present themselves that will be enlightening to you, but you needn't worry about uncovering information that's too much to handle. You'll be taking a straightforward inventory of your character the way a shopkeeper inventories goods in a store. It's a necessary part of your experiment in giving your poor, weary willpower a rest and in using love's power from here on. There are many ways to take personal inventory, but the clear and basic procedure suggested in the book *Alcoholics Anonymous* is time-tested for success. The recommendation there is for a three-part inventory covering resentment, fear, and sex.

The resentment list has three columns: one for the person or institution resented, a second for what he, she, or it did to cause the resentment, and a third for how that affects you. As an example, you might write that you resent (first column) your sister because (second column) she says you ought to lose weight, which affects (third column) your self-esteem.

The resentment inventory is both healing and informative. In column two, where you're able to write about precisely what your resentments are, you're also recognizing feelings that you may have denied for a long time. This is certainly healthy, but in itself it's not enough. To be free of resentment, it's necessary to see what's going on inside you, thus the reason for having column three. *Alcoholics Anonymous* cites self-esteem, pride, sexual relations, and finances as those areas of our lives most likely to be the wounded parties when we're holding resentment.

Fear underlies a great many of the difficulties in all these areas. As you notice what comes out over and over in the third column, you'll be getting to know yourself much better.

The second part of the inventory is a list of fears. What are you afraid of? A sample fear list might look something like this.

- Losing my job
- Getting cancer
- Being fat forever
- Being hungry
- Flying
- Getting old

Whatever your fear, write it down. Keep writing as long as things occur to you. Nothing is too petty. If it comes to mind, it's in your heart, so put it in your inventory.

Fears are also telling. The sample list shows insecurities around issues of health, safety, and finances. Some people have deeply embedded fears, which may require special work in a therapeutic setting. But many fear patterns can be traded for a faith response as soon as we decide to do it. Looking at the fears straight on starts the process.

The final part of the inventory concerns sexuality. Look at your past and present relationships and write about them. *Alcoholics Anonymous* suggests you answer the following questions:

Where had we been selfish, dishonest, or inconsiderate?
Whom had we hurt?
Did we unjustifiably arouse jealousy, suspicion, or bitterness?
Where were we at fault and what should we have done instead?
We subjected each relation to this test—Was it selfish or not?

You may find it helpful to add to these such additional queries as:

When have I allowed myself to be hurt?
Have I settled for sex when I was looking for love?
Do I accept myself as a sexual being?
Is there balance in my sexuality—that is, can I both enjoy and respect it?

Your answers are to provide insights into who you are, not provoke feelings of guilt. This is an inventory, not the Inquisition.

If you do all three parts and you still feel that there's something missing, write whatever else comes to mind. And get a complete picture by topping off your inventory with a list of the things you admire and appreciate about yourself. False modesty is no good here. There are many splendid things about you. Write at least ten. Better still: fifty.

Then share the whole thing with another person. If you're in a Twelve Step group, you can do this with someone who has done it already. Otherwise, choose someone whom you trust to listen without judgment and accept you just as you are. Revealing the nooks and crannies of your soul to someone else—ideally someone who has seen and revealed nooks and crannies of his own soul—brings a tremendous sense of peace. Some people feel that they're truly a part of life for the first time after sharing their true selves with another person, as well as with themselves and with the God of their understanding.

As we continue with the Twelve Steps' suggestions for cleaning up the past, Step 6 discusses our readiness to be without the character defects found in our inventories. It's counter-intuitive that we may want to hang on to shortcomings that have caused us pain and lured us into the kitchen. The fact is, we do often cling to them, just as we've clung to abusing food. There was a time when we needed that food because we didn't have anything better. Now we do.

Similarly, we no longer need many of the defects of character that we had thought were necessary to make it in the world. When our lives are based on spiritual principles, we can prosper without dishonesty or manipulation because we are able to accept success as Love reaching out to us. We can meet our needs without interfering with others meeting their needs because we'll realize there's enough fulfillment to go around. And we can feel satisfied with the food we need to be healthy and full of energy without looking to extra or inferior food that promises satisfaction but only bogs us down.

When we ask that troublesome parts of our personalities be taken away, we find that most aren't so much removed as redeemed. A pushy personality can become an outgoing, assertive one. Hypersensitivity becomes motivated sensitivity to the plight

A Mental Makeover

. . . .

Unproductive, negative thoughts can be turned into powerful, productive ones. Here are some examples of typical sub-zero self-talk and the respective Point Zero responses.

SUB-ZERO THINKING	POINT ZERO RESPONSES
I don't measure up.	I am adequate and more than adequate.
I don't belong here.	I am at home in my life and in my world.
Other people have their lives together.	I refuse to compare how my life feels to how their lives look.
There's some secret to happiness, but I don't have it.	I discover something to be happy about every day.
If I could lose weight (or stop purging), my life would be in order.	I live in an orderly way at my present weight.
If I didn't manage everyone and everything, there would be chaos.	I take care of my own life and leave the rest to God.
If you knew the real me, you wouldn't like me.	I am a likable person through and through.
Things have been too good; I'm due for something awful.	Things are good and I am grateful.
Whatever it is, it's my fault (or your fault).	My focus is on solving the problem, not assigning blame.
I'm afraid of what will happen.	I live in the safety of the present moment.
I don't know what to do.	I do the next thing indicated.
I can't keep up the façade.	I am who and what I am.
If you would change, I could.	I make the changes that are right for me regardless of anyone else's behavior.
I know what to do, but I'm doing just the opposite.	I know what to do and, alone or with help, I do it.
I can't (try, start, risk, succeed), so I won't.	I can (try, start, risk, succeed), and I'm doing it.
I'm tired and I haven't done anything.	I have plenty of energy to do what is mine to do.
If I'm not perfect, I'm a failure.	I am a perfect human being and perfect human beings have flaws.
Nobody else is like me.	I am a member of the human family.
I'm a special case.	I'm a special person.

of other people, other creatures, and perhaps a heightened appreciation for art or nature. Low self-esteem can morph into humble self-appreciation.

That word *humble* can have a red flag attached, and since Step 7 is worded "Humbly asked [God] to remove our shortcomings," this word deserves some attention. We confuse it with humiliation, which food addicts have so often suffered, instead of humility, of which most people, fat or thin, addicted or not, could handle a hearty helping. Humility implies being who we are, not something other than that. And since we are already magnificent in our very humanness, why would anyone want to be more? Perhaps it's because we've often believed ourselves to be much less.

I like the status of humility conferred on Wilbur the Pig in the children's classic *Charlotte's Web* by E. B. White. In it, Wilbur is spared from slaughter because his buddy, a literate spider named Charlotte, writes about him, by seemingly miraculous means, in her web. First come the accolades: Wilbur is "some pig," then he is "terrific" and "radiant." Charlotte's last weaving for her porcine companion is that he is "humble." That may have been the highest tribute of all.

Steps 8 and 9 on the Twelve Step path discuss making peace with other people or with ourselves regarding them. By going back to the inventory, you'll see names of people you've hurt or with whom you've had some discord. Without assigning the role of villain to either you or them, you'll see that these are people with whom there is outstanding acrimony that keeps you from balancing your life, the way that checks too long outstanding can keep you from balancing your account. Step 8 involves listing those people and Step 9 involves making amends to those you've harmed, if that's possible, "except when to do so would injure them or others."

There are plenty of reasons for wanting to bypass this step. You could say:

- More people have harmed me than I've ever harmed.
- He deserved what he got for what he did. (She did, too.)
- That creep is out of my life and I like it that way.
- I don't want to dredge up old dirt.
- It's easier to hold the grudge.
- This has nothing to do with how I eat.

I understand these objections and they may have validity—except for the last one. As human beings, human relationships motivate us more than any other factor beyond survival itself. We can deny their importance, but they are important nonetheless. Relations with other people have a great deal to do with what, when, how, and why a person with a food problem eats.

Be clear on what making amends entails. It's not groveling before another person, begging forgiveness, or re-establishing a partnership or friendship that has run its course. It is instead to amend the current, unsatisfactory situation.

Person-to-person amends are like Amendments to the Constitution. The people who drafted the original document didn't look at it afterward and say, "Oh, we left out freedom of speech and freedom of the press. Too bad." No, they amended what they had done with the Bill of Rights. That's what we need to do in our dealings with other people. We can amend (change, add to) our attitude or behavior toward them to make the relationship better.

Sometimes the best relationship is no relationship. That's fine. Your willingness to make each one the best that it can be is the goal. In the cases in which making an amend could honestly hurt that person or someone else, you can amend the situation within yourself. That is, you can choose to genuinely forgive the other person for his or her part in the situation, and grant yourself the same courtesy. If this is someone you don't see anymore, it may not be appropriate to seek this person out. Nevertheless, if you should run into him at some point, you would have already instigated a healing of the past.

In some cases, amends can mean a simple apology. Others require paying a monetary debt or making good on a promise. The process also calls for putting your own name on top of your list and becoming fast friends with yourself. As you treat each situation in turn, you'll find those "outstanding checks" coming in, and you'll be able to go to a new bank with free checking and lots of ATMs. In other words, your life will be richer so your food won't have to be. Your life will be simpler so your food can be, too.

Expand Your Comfort Zone

There was once a widow who was always happy. She was at home in the parlors of the wealthy and titled who sought her counsel, and in the hovels of beggars to whom she brought cheer as well as bread and firewood. She delighted in the laughter of children and the ramblings of the aged, in autumn leaves and spring flowers, in praying and in dancing.

In her town there lived a sorcerer. He was not an evil man, but he was selfish and used to getting his own way. He asked the widow for her daughter's hand in marriage. Now, she remembered something of marital bliss, and not wanting her daughter to wed an old man, refused him. The sorcerer was angry and sought retribution.

First he brought fevered sickness upon the woman, but she still had the joy of her daughter's sweet voice and her many friends to nurse her back to health. Next the sorcerer condemned her to poverty. She and her daughter learned to forage for herbs and wild berries. On this frugal fare, the woman's face lost most of its lines and an annoying bit of rheumatism left her.

Further angered by the thwarting of his revenge, the sorcerer thought long on the perfect spell. "This one she shall not overcome!" he vowed. Under the final curse, the woman was to have no peace, whatever the circumstances. She felt unfit to converse with the rich but too well-bred to associate with the poor, so she was lonely. Rain was too cold for her and sun too hot, so she stayed indoors. Work seemed drudgery and play foolishness, so there was nothing to fill her hours. The woman was happy no longer.

She begged mercy of the sorcerer. "You have taken from me my most precious gift, the ability to be happy in any company and in any occupation. This was the greatest bequest I had to leave my daughter. Without it, I see no other way than to take her life and my own."

The sorcerer's heart was moved to pity. "Woman, I see that what I seek is not your daughter's hand but her mother's secret." He lifted the curse and learned from the woman how to find contentment in every circumstance. And if you go to that town today, some will tell you that there is more to the story, that indeed the woman and the sorcerer were joined in marriage and lived many happy years together.

Food Facts for Point Zero

. . . .

- Eating everything on your plate will not help a single starving child. Throwing away food that you don't need is not terrible. If the food is good for your dog, feed it to the dog. If not, feed it to the Earth via a compost pile.

- It's possible to get a fix from not eating just as it is from eating. Do you get high from dieting or missing meals? Look at your behavior around food. The goal is balance, to get food into its proper place in your life as a whole. That will mean diminishing its importance overall and not looking to food, either more or less than you need, to feel better.

- You can prepare a meal without eating half of it in the process. At first you may wish to cook from recipes so you'll know the seasoning is right without tasting. If you do need to taste, do so at the end of the cooking process. A tiny taste will tell you all you need to know.

- If some food situations are particularly problematic, you can ask those around you for help. As an example, if you've gotten into the habit of finishing off your children's leftovers while you clear the table, make getting the dishes to the sink or dishwasher their job, not yours. Eventually, that kind of temptation may not matter, but as long as it does, give yourself a break.

- There's no magical food that will "melt pounds" or take away your appetite forever or anything like that. Appreciate what's seemingly magical about food: that it can fuel one very important organism—yours. If your relationship with food has been awful, approach it with an attitude that's more awe-filled.

- Food is neutral, like water. Water is a necessity, but it can also flood your basement, shrink your best pants, or even take your life. Similarly, food becomes a problem when it's misused or ill-chosen. For this reason, your focus needs to be first on your life, then on your food.

- Wanting to lose weight is not the same thing as wanting to stop eating for a fix. A heartfelt desire to live fix-free carries in itself tremendous power because it implies a willingness to live by the laws of nature and, if you will, of God. There's nothing wrong with desiring to lose weight simply to have a slimmer body, but spiritually it's about on par with desiring a trip to Las Vegas.

- You can say no to any food offered to you by any person on this planet. If that person is offended, there's a problem, but the problem isn't yours.

The woman in this little tale had a wide comfort zone. She found acceptance from everyone because she offered it to everyone, and she found delight in myriad activities because she looked for it in all of them. My friend Rita is like that. She loves opera, but she listens to country music on car trips so she can feel like a trucker. She knows about a million subjects, is convinced that she has never met an uninteresting person, and treats the world as if it were an amusement park to which she has a season pass. Rita has taught me a lot about comfort zones.

We all have one—that place or set of circumstances in which we feel safe, comfortable, and unthreatened. We stray from its center in situations that are unfamiliar or with which we have negative past associations. In these cases we tend to feel out of place; we may be uncomfortable with not knowing what to do or what's expected of us. It's only natural to feel more at ease in a friendly, familiar environment with people we know well than in an unfamiliar place with strangers. Nevertheless, when we're grounded in the love-based life, when we start each day from Point Zero, we carry an expandable comfort zone with us.

When you bring these principles to life by living them, you'll find that your serenity will no longer need to come from personal charm, although you may be charming, or from knowing the social graces, although you may be graced with every one of them. It will instead come as a gift from your indwelling Higher Power. You'll be able to talk with your boss or a subordinate, the President or some freckled friend of your ten-year-old, and be genuinely interested in that person and genuinely secure in yourself. You'll be looking across at people instead of up or down at any of them.

The fine line between a frightening situation and an exciting one will blur, and your increasingly positive outlook will choose excitement over anxiety every time. Beyond this, however, you'll find that your need for excitement will decrease and your preference for serenity will grow. Because you'll become proficient at getting what you need, more and more serenity will become available to you.

Start where you are right now. Perhaps your comfort zone seems small. You may think that almost no place on Earth is truly safe unless you're armored with food or protective layers of fat. Don't despair if you feel that you're starting from the bottom. Start. Create your own safe, nurturing, binge-free, guilt-free comfort zone. At first, this may be a private spot just for you. Then you can gradually expand it to include one other person you trust, then others.

Your comfort zone may well be much broader than this at the outset, but some places or activities may still seem unsafe: supermarkets, interpersonal confrontations, speaking before groups. Allow your comfort zone to grow. If you need to buy groceries, talk with a co-worker about a potentially volatile topic, or give a twenty-minute talk, use the same techniques you did for sitting with your feelings—only this time you're accepting outer situations in the same way that you accepted inner ones. In this case, instead of quietly being with your feelings, take appropriate action, regardless of your feelings.

As you incorporate more and more honest living, honest eating, facing feelings, and letting go of the past into the framework of your life, your comfort zone will expand automatically. You'll find yourself in possession of a degree of poise that may surprise you. You might attribute it to a new haircut or taking vitamins or losing ten pounds, and if that helps—well, here's to haircuts. But as you encourage the flowering of your spiritual self, you'll come to see that that's the key to your becoming more and more relaxed with whatever the day presents.

No one has nonstop equanimity, but yours can increase exponentially as you come to accept yourself more and more. As you do that, you'll also come to accept what's going on around you for precisely what it is at the moment, even those things that need to be changed. The more you're able to accept the way things are, the larger your comfort zone will become. This in no way means tolerating abuse or settling for less than you need. On the contrary, it means finding a centered spot in the midst of any circumstance. From that zone of comfort, from Point Zero, you can enjoy the positive and deal wisely and rationally with any negative elements that present themselves.

When my daughter was in kindergarten, I commented to her that a certain minor difficulty was really a blessing. "Disguised or the other kind?" she wanted to know. There's a place where the disguised ones are as valuable as the others, and blessings of every sort abound. That place is Point Zero. You may be there now as you read this book. If not, know that you're on your way.

CHAPTER FOUR

LOOKING IN, REACHING OUT

I spent years of my life looking for balance. I wanted the scale to balance on one number rather than another, but that balance eluded me until a more important balance was struck. That's the balance between my inner world and my outer one. In active food addiction, one of these invariably outweighs the other. Often I was caught up with work, other people, and frenzied activity, thereby avoiding who I really was. At other times, I stayed alone as much as possible, shielded with food, books, and TV. The built-in isolation of eating for a fix kept me separated from both the richness of my interior world and of the world around me.

If you relate to that kind of separation, you can rest easy knowing that with every day you live fix-free, you'll gently come more fully into the stream of life in a balanced way. Conversely, as you invite that fullness of life into your own experience, you'll find that abstinence from unhealthful eating gradually becomes natural and effortless. The task at hand has two parts: first, to look within through self-study, meditation, and prayer, then to reach out to others in friendship and service.

Life is filled with such inner and outer dualities. Creativity, for example, needs an idea (internal) and expression (external). Each depends on the other. Artists don't lose their talents when they express them. On the contrary, every poem or painting refines, perfects, and intensifies the creative capacity of the person responsible for it. Along with your growing realization of your spiritual nature, your positive feelings and exuberance will actually increase as you express them in all you do.

Understandably, a lot of people regard spirituality as optional at best because it appears to have to do only with intangibles. For addicts, however, those intangibles can get solid pretty fast. We require an active, sometimes intense, spiritual practice in order to have a life worth living. Our spirituality provides us with the wherewithal to deal with food, people, and problems just as surely as our work provides us with money for paying bills and going shopping. Declining a spiritual life would do to our recovery what declining an income source would do to our buying power.

You may already acknowledge your spirituality. To bring it to bear on your food situation could mean simply expanding that acknowledgment, coming to realize that food addiction affects the soul as well as the body and that it's important enough to take to your God. Or perhaps you don't buy all this spirituality stuff. Self-examination may seem unnecessary and prayer ridiculous. Why pray if there's no one to hear? Why share and risk rejection? I think that we look inside when we're tired of living with a stranger. We pray when we're tired of living alone, and we share because we're grateful that we're no longer tired.

You see, spirituality is like food and exercise. If you don't eat, you can survive on fat reserves but not indefinitely. If you don't exercise, your muscle tone will last for a while but not for long. Going within provides you with spiritual food; giving to others is your spiritual workout. Their relationship is symbiotic.

Specializing in Transformation

There's still another difference between what we've done together so far and the other approaches that you've probably taken in an attempt to change the way you eat. Where diets and their ilk focus on food, we're focusing on you and your relationship with the spiritual power within you that specializes in transformation.

That goes far beyond the mere restructuring of your body. When a physical change happens without the involvement of the rest of your being, it's doomed from the outset. It's no wonder that ninety percent of the people who lose twenty-five pounds or more are said to regain it within two years. They don't realize that the body is, ultimately, a reflection—a reflection of what's going on inside: emotionally, intellectually, and spiritually. A physical body of the size you fancy hasn't a chance of staying that way without the support of your heart, mind, and soul.

Weight loss by itself is like winning the lottery. It's terrific, but many lottery winners, like weight losers, wake up at some point where they started, wondering what happened. What happened is that the recently rich aren't always able to develop the attitudes (emotion), knowledge (intellect), and/or consciousness (spirit) necessary to maintain prosperity. And the suddenly svelte usually lack the attitudes, knowledge, and/or consciousness to maintain a body of pleasing proportions. (Attitude and consciousness are far more important than knowledge. With the right attitude and consciousness, you'll get the knowledge you need. You can, however, be a literal information bank on fitness, nutrition, and pop psychology, yet still be caught in the morass of compulsive eating.)

Both lottery winners and weight losers experience a change in form—net worth or gross poundage—but transformation is more than that. Dr. Wayne Dyer, who does a lot of work with this idea, defines transformation as "going beyond form." That's what your love-powered release of weight will be: a going beyond the form (this size or that, a larger waist measurement or a smaller one) to become the sort of person whose desires, preferences, and practices sustain a healthy, attractive body as a matter of course.

You've already realized that you can no more control your weight than you can control your grown children or the commodities market. Instead, you need to become someone for whom weight control is no longer an issue. This proceeds from the inside out. You've built a strong foundation while following the suggestions in the previous chapters. Now you'll be looking at ways to guarantee daily renewal of the spiritual fitness necessary to keep food addiction at bay. That guarantee depends on keeping your life in ethical order, developing a viable relationship with the God of your understanding, and being of service to others as you put your entire life on a spiritual basis.

Remember that *spiritual*, as we're using the word, can be defined as *transformational*. It certainly can imply religious convictions, but for the purpose of leaving your addiction behind you, generic spirituality works just as well. Your personal spirituality can be nurtured on a continuing basis with the final three of the Twelve

Steps. The first of these, Step 10, states: "Continued to take personal inventory, and when we were wrong, promptly admitted it."

Routine Maintenance

Think of your character as a car. The moral inventory in Step 4 was a major tune-up; this ongoing, daily inventory is routine maintenance. When you take care of your car, you don't have to worry about driving it. When you take care of your life, you don't have to worry about living it.

Because we learn from mistakes, we're bound to make them as long as we're alive. We can't afford to deny them, rationalize them, or wallow in them. That's what ongoing inventory is about. The book *Alcoholics Anonymous* gives explicit instructions for how to go about this: "We continue to watch for selfishness, dishonesty, resentment, and fear. When these crop up, we ask God at once to remove them. We discuss them with someone immediately and make amends quickly if we have harmed anyone. Then we resolutely turn our thoughts to someone we can help."

This is gratis guilt prevention. A mistake is like an accidental spill. Guilt is the stain that develops if it isn't cleaned up. Making instant amends most profoundly benefits us, but it also does wonders for our relations with others. We don't allow minor slights and misunderstandings to escalate into major ones. We don't allow the time to elapse in which our difficulties with another person could be taken to gossip court and tried by a jury of our peers.

Many people find it helpful to take a nightly mini-inventory in addition to their daily lookout for selfishness, dishonesty, resentment, and fear. This inventory is a mental scan of the preceding waking hours to detect any unresolved disharmony or discomfort. Sometimes all you need to do here is forgive yourself and go to bed. Perhaps you'll want to offer a situation to your Higher Power or run it past a person you trust. If something needs to be done tomorrow about what you said or did today, make a note to that effect in your mind or in your journal, and tuck it away for the night.

Quality Time with Your Higher Power

Before you go to sleep, spend a few quiet minutes with yourself and your Higher Power. Have another quiet time in the morning before the demands of the day take all your attention. This is when you indulge yourself in the peacefulness of prayer and meditation. Certainly you can "pray without ceasing" in your thoughts and actions overall and maintain the Buddhists' attitude of *mindfulness*, a meditative appreciation of every moment as you go through your day. But setting aside some minutes specifically devoted to your inner life is necessary, too. You have quality time with your children. This is quality time with yourself—and your God.

The Twelve Steps discuss this in Step 11, which says, "Sought through prayer and meditation to improve our conscious contact with God as we understood Him, praying only for knowledge of His will for us and the power to carry that out."

For many people, this is a compelling invitation just as it's written, but if the word *God* doesn't give you feelings of warmth and peace, use another name or another image. Change "His will" to "Her will" if that, as the Quakers would say, better "speaks to your condition."

A recovering alcoholic who writes anonymously as Rachel V. addresses this eloquently in her book *A Woman Like You*: "In [Alcoholics Anonymous] meetings now, I say that I'm promiscuous with God. I call on everyone: the Blessed Mother, the Lord Buddha, God the Father, Jesus Christ, Tara, the Holy Ghost, my grandmother, Inanna, Kuan Yin, Isis, Ishtar, Kali, Sophia, the Shekina, anybody and everybody. I need all the help I can get. I'm sure that God understands. My life is evidence."

Striking a balance between our inner and outer worlds can reveal that kind of evidence in any of our lives. Prayer and meditation symbolize this balance, because with them we *reach out* to a Higher Power by *looking within* to the place in ourselves where that Power resides. A legend from India tells of the upset the gods experienced after they created humans. They were afraid that this cocky species would discover divine truth and that people would then become gods themselves. To avoid being overtaken by upstarts, the gods tried to figure out where they might hide the truth out of humans' reach. If they hid it in the treetops, a person could climb there. If they hid it at the bottom of the sea, someone would dive down to discover it. The cleverest of the gods finally suggested, "Let us hide the truth deep inside every individual. That is the one place they'll never look."

Well, sometimes we do. That's what prayer and meditation are about. Basically, prayer is talking to God and meditation is letting God answer. There's no single right way to do either one. If you follow a religious teaching, there's likely to be a wealth of information about prayer and meditation within your own tradition. As you explore it with renewed appreciation, you're apt to see a depth and beauty there that may have eluded you before.

If you don't have such a tradition to draw on (or you have one but you're not interested in going back there), you can still rest easy knowing that prayer comes naturally to human beings as long as we don't get caught up in trivialities such as "thee" and "thou" and "ah-men" versus "a-men." If prayer is new to you, if you haven't tried it lately, or if you're feeling inhibited or skeptical about it, here are some suggestions.

How to Talk to Your Higher Power

Talk with your Higher Power the way you'd talk with a trusted friend. Don't bother thee-ing and thou-ing. Just talk—silently is fine. Share what's going on with you. If you feel foolish doing it, talk about that, too. You can share anything—even if it seems petty or you think that God would disapprove. The loving God you're coming to know doesn't disapprove of you.

- Read or commit to memory a couple of prayers that appeal to you. Think about the words and what they mean.
- In the morning, offer your day to God. Ask for help with your eating and for the decisions you'll make during the next twenty-four hours. Ask to remember in the midst of all your activities that you're no longer by yourself.
- Write to God. Put your thoughts, feelings, concerns, and delights down in a notebook or journal.
- Start a prayer list or a prayer box. Put the names of people who are on your mind or situations beyond your control on a list in your notebook or in

A Prayer Primer

. . . .

Someone once told me that it's important to have prayers, poems, and uplifting quotations filed away in my memory bank because there'd be times I'd be alone with only what was in my mind. If I'd stored away words of beauty and inspiration, they'd be there for me. I've found that to be true. Some of those that serve me well are included here. Feel free to choose from these (many of which will be familiar to you) or find your own. You never need to use prewritten prayers in order to talk with your Higher Power, but they do make good company.

THE SERENITY PRAYER

God, grant me the serenity to accept the things I cannot change,
The courage to change the things I can,
And the wisdom to know the difference.
(*This prayer, which many refer to as the AA prayer and which is, in fact, used by most, and perhaps all, Twelve Step fellowships, is the slightly adapted form of an unnamed prayer first written in the 1930s by theologian Reinhold Niebuhr.*)

THE PRAYER FOR PROTECTION
by James Dillet Freeman
First published by Unity School of Christianity

The light of God surrounds me.
The love of God enfolds me.
The power of God protects me.
The presence of God watches over me.
Wherever I am, God is.

THE LORD'S PRAYER

Our Father who art in heaven, Hallowed be thy name. Thy kingdom come. Thy will be done on Earth, as it is in heaven. Give us this day our daily bread. And forgive us our debts, as we forgive our debtors. And lead us not into temptation, but deliver us from evil: For thine is the kingdom, and the power, and the glory, for ever.

A SIKH DEVOTION
from the Asa Ki Var

Wonderful Thy word, wonderful Thy knowledge; Wonderful Thy creatures, wonderful their species; Wonderful their forms, wonderful their colors; Wonderful the animals which wander naked; Wonderful Thy wind, wonderful Thy water; Wonderful Thy fire which sporteth wondrously; Wonderful the earth, wonderful the sources of production; Wonderful the pleasures to which mortals are attached; Wonderful is meeting, wonderful parting from Thee; Wonderful is hunger, wonderful repletion; Wonderful Thy praises, wonderful Thy eulogies; Wonderful the desert, wonderful the road; Wonderful Thy nearness, wonderful Thy remoteness; Wonderful to behold Thee present. Beholding these wonderful things I remain wondering.

A HINDU PRAYER

Lead me from the unreal to the Real.
Lead me from darkness to Light.
Lead me from death to the knowledge of Immortality.
May the entire world be happy.

A PRAYER OF ST. FRANCIS

Lord, make me an instrument of your peace.
Where there is hatred, let me bring love.
Where there is injury, let me bring pardon.
Where there is discord, let me bring harmony.
Where there is error, let me bring truth.
Where there is doubt, let me bring faith.
Where there is despair, let me bring hope.
Where there is darkness, let me bring light.
Where there is sadness, let me bring joy.
Lord, grant that I may seek not so much
To be comforted as to comfort,
To be understood as to understand,
To be loved as to love.
For it is in seeking that we find.
It is in forgiving that we are forgiven.
It is in dying to the things of self
That we are born to Eternal Life.

AN ANTHROPOSOPHICAL PRAYER

by Rudolf Steiner

May the events that seek me come unto me.
May I receive them through the
Father's ground of peace on which we walk.
May the people who seek me come unto me.
May I receive them with an understanding heart through the
Christ's stream of love in which we live.
May the spirits that seek me come unto me.
May I receive them with a clean soul through the Healing Spirit's light by which we see.

THE TWENTY-THIRD PSALM

The Lord is my shepherd; I shall not want.
He maketh me to lie down in green pastures; he leadeth me beside the still waters.
He restoreth my soul; he leadeth me in the paths of righteousness for his name's sake.
Yea, though I walk through the valley of the shadow of death,
I will fear no evil: for thou art with me; thy rod and thy staff they comfort me.
Thou preparest a table before me in the presence of mine enemies; thou anointest my
    head with oil; my cup runneth over.
Surely goodness and mercy shall follow me all the days of my life: and I will dwell in the
    house of the Lord forever.

ON PRAYER

from *The Prophet*, by Kahlil Gibran

Our God, who art our winged self, it is thy will in us that willeth.
It is thy desire in us that desireth.
It is thy urge in us that would turn our nights, which are thine, into days which are
    thine also.
We cannot ask thee for aught, for thou knowest our needs before they are born in us:
Thou art our need;
And in giving us more of thyself thou givest us all.

THE GREAT INVOCATION
by Alice Bailey

From the point of Love within the Heart of God
Let love stream forth into the hearts of men.
May Christ return to Earth.
From the center where the Will of God is known
Let purpose guide the little wills of men—
The purpose which the Masters know and serve.
From the center which we call the race of men
Let the Plan of Love and Light work out
And may it seal the door where evil dwells.
Let Light and Love and Power restore the Plan on Earth.

NATIVE AMERICAN PRAYER

Now Talking God
With your feet I walk.
I walk with your limbs.
I carry forth your body.
For me your mind thinks;
Your voice speaks for me.
Beauty is before me
And beauty behind me;
Above and below me hovers the beautiful:
I am surrounded by it,
I am immersed in it.
In my youth I am aware of it.
And in old age I shall walk quietly
The beautiful trail.

a small box or jar. Think of these names or situations when you have some quiet time.

- Pray with your voice, your body, and your creativity. Song, dance, and art can be powerful prayers.
- Spend time in nature. Reverence is an effortless part of that.

- Pray with someone else. This can be uncomfortable if you're not used to it. If you persist, however, you'll find a special relationship developing not only between you and your Higher Power, but between you and the person with whom you're praying.

- Explore affirmative prayer. Affirmative prayer is aligning your thoughts with God's through statements of divine truth. It's a way of opening yourself to the blessings you may have been ignoring, but which are nevertheless immediately available to you. Affirmations are positive statements like, "God loves me, so I love and care for my body."

Most of us are used to praying *for* things, even bargaining for something like, "Get me out of this one, and I'll do volunteer work twenty-two hours a week for the rest of my life." We've treated God like a celestial Santa Claus, and when we don't get all the goodies on our list, we assume that prayer doesn't work or even that there is no God. It doesn't take much logic, however, to see that praying for things or for specific outcomes couldn't work in an orderly universe. I could pray for my side to win the war or the football game and you could pray for your side to win. Is God supposed to play favorites?

Or someone could pray to lose weight while slurping a *grande* mocha with extra whipped cream. That's asking for a circumvention of natural law and is about as absurd as praying, "You know, God, I'm really sick of all this gravitational pull. How about letting me float around fifty or sixty feet above ground for a while?"

Besides, praying for things and automatically getting them would mean avoiding the lessons we're here to learn. Learning from life is as inviolable a principle as the laws governing gravity or the metabolizing of that mocha. This may well be why Step 11 includes the phrase, "praying only for knowledge of [God's] will for us and the power to carry that out." Now *that* can be horrifying. It's fine to let God have the cycles of nature and the orbiting of planets, but when it comes to *my* life, *my* relationships, and certainly the size of *my* jeans, I ought to know what's best. But you know what? I didn't know what was best all the time and I still don't.

Of course, I can set goals, make choices, and steer my life in the direction that seems to be the proper one based on my intelligence, experience, and common sense. But intelligence, experience, and common sense aren't enough for a truly successful life. It also takes uncommon sense, intuition, and sometimes nothing short of divine providence. All prayers are answered, but sometimes when we pray for what we want, the answer is "No." When we pray instead for the will of the God that loves us no matter what, the answer is always "Yes," always right, and always best in the long run.

When I was still doing periodic binge eating, someone told me to stop praying for anything, even to get over my food addiction. "I only pray to be of service," she said. "Then I get everything else." I didn't trust that until I began to see it work in my own life. First, I stopped praying to lose weight. I prayed instead to live in keeping with the laws of life. The prayer was answered as the foods I selected changed and I started showing up at the gym on a fairly regular basis. Obesity cannot coexist with that lifestyle. I didn't have to pray to lose weight or work to lose weight. I prayed for God's will and, as my friend had also discovered, I got everything else.

Praying for God's will is not ignoring our problems and distresses. *The Twelve Steps and Twelve Traditions of Overeaters Anonymous* explains, "Clearly, if we are to develop a vital relationship with a Higher Power, we'll need to bring into our prayers all the things that concern us. We pray about these things, not so we can get our way but so we can bring our will regarding them into alignment with God's will." Lasting peace of mind and the ability to live fix-free depend upon that alignment.

Inner Listening

But how do we come to know what God's will for us is? Well, we ask for it in prayer—then wait for an answer. This brings us to meditation: the state of mental stillness in which the still, small voice may be heard. Sometimes called *contemplation* or *contemplative prayer*, meditation is found in all religious traditions and physicians and psychologists recommend it for stress reduction. Simply stated, meditation is mental focusing. The object of that focus may be a word or syllable, an object such as a flower or candle flame, a phrase from a prayer or a scripture, or simply your own breath as you sit quietly observing your inhalations and exhalations—breathing in, breathing out, one breath at a time, no hurry, no worry, nothing to do but sit, watch, wait, breathe, and listen.

An easy beginning meditation is to count your breaths. Count "one" on the inhalation, and use a word such as *love, peace,* or *shalom* to mark the exhalation. Count "one," *peace*; "two," *peace*; "three," *peace*; "four," *peace,* and so on until you reach "ten." Then start again. (If you hit seventeen before you realize you've passed ten, gently bring yourself back to one. You're doing fine.)

When your mind wanders to what's on your desk at work, bring it back: "one," *peace*; "two," *peace*; "three," *peace*. . . . When your mind wanders to what to wear to the party this weekend, bring it back: "four," *peace*; "five," *peace*; "six," *peace*. . . . When your mind wanders to world affairs, your father's surgery, or your teenager's SAT scores, bring it back and focus: "seven," *peace*; "eight," *peace*; "nine", *peace*; "ten," *peace*. . . . Then start again: Inhale "one," exhale *peace*; inhale "two," exhale *peace*. . . .

Do it for at least ten minutes in the morning. Doing twenty minutes in both morning and evening would be ideal, but even a little meditation beats none at all. Your relief from addictive eating or obsessive weight control will come with living in the love you're offered by love's very source. There's no substitute for connecting with that source voluntarily, regularly, and repeatedly. This may seem like a lot to do, but after you've made a place in your life for prayer and meditation, you'll wonder what you ever did without them. By reading about them and talking with people who already practice these spiritual disciplines, you'll devise your own routine for getting your much-needed inner nourishment.

Your personal meditation practice will fit your schedule and your temperament. I, for example, am not a marathon meditator. There are times when I find it boring and would rather get on with the real highlights of life, like bringing in the newspaper and feeding the cat. I don't hear voices, see visions, levitate, or get any other noteworthy amusement from praying and meditating, nor would I want to. But I'm more peaceful than I used to be—and less afraid. My life works pretty well, and right now I'm thinking about writing this page instead of thinking about something to eat. I believe that a great deal of the credit for this goes to the little bit of silence I take for myself virtually every day.

I start my day by recalling, even before I open my eyes, the realities that govern my life as a food addict: I cannot control food—that's the Higher Power's department; I renew my commitment to letting that Power deal with my life and my food for the upcoming twenty-four hours. Once I'm officially awake, I try to get to prayer and meditation right away. It doesn't always work out this way, but letting too many other things interfere can delete quiet time altogether.

Some people have a special chair or even a special room for meditation. I'm less formal. I usually sit up in bed Indian-style and start by writing in my journal. If there's something on my mind, it gets prayed out in pen and ink. If I'm feeling sorry for myself, I make a list of things I have to be grateful for. If the day ahead seems complicated, I write out my supposed obligations and see which of them really need to be done and which don't. In this way I clear my brain just as orators clear their throats.

Then I read something centering, usually a selection from a daily devotional book such as *For Today* from Overeaters Anonymous, or from *Daily Word* or *Science of Mind*, magazines comprised of short, inspirational readings for every day of the month. Then I close my eyes, check to see that I'm sitting in some semblance of erectness (I want to be alert for this), and allow my mind to mull over the words I've just read. When my thoughts go off in other directions, I bring them back to those words, to their ideas. Sometimes I need more structure and do the breath-counting meditation instead. In either case I finish with a prayer to do God's will that day. All of this takes about thirty minutes. Sometimes I cut it short. My best days are when I don't.

Spawning Miracles

At night I thank my Higher Power for the day. Some days have been filled with so many surprises and successes I'm over the moon about them. Other times I do well to say thanks that my food was OK and that the day is over. I sometimes read a little nighttime thought from a book I like, but I don't have a bona fide bedtime meditation. At least I don't yet—but life is so much richer thanks to the modicum of inward turning I do already, surely any addition would be all to the good. Still,

To Keep a Journal

. . . .

There are many ways to pray and meditate. You can be in your house or your synagogue, on the beach or on the bus. You can pray and meditate while kneeling or walking, in the lotus position on the floor or in your favorite chair. And you can express yourself to yourself and to God through silent thoughts, spoken words, or in writing in your journal.

A spiritual journal entails much more than keeping a diary or calendar, although it can incorporate those functions. The real purpose of a spiritual journal is to facilitate your inner growth. How it does this depends upon you and what you want to achieve, but a journal can be used in any of the following ways.

- Write in it in the morning to become grounded in the day at hand. There's something about writing today's date that implies a commitment to the nonrefundable span of time you'll have to spend during this day.

- Record your food, either as a flexible plan for the day ahead or in the evening as a record of the gift of sane eating that you received.

- Describe your feelings when you're feeling a lot of anything, even if you can't label those feelings right away.

- Write about decisions you have to make. List the pros and cons of your choices. This will help to clear your thinking process.

- Write down what you need to do for the day. If there are forty-four things to do in a twenty-four-hour day, laugh. Then make cuts.

- Write out affirmations. It's fine to speak statements of universal truth, but when you write them, especially if you do it several times a day for a month or so, they become *your* statements of personal truth.

- Write letters to God (instant delivery, quicker than texting).

- Write down ideas that you see or hear and want to internalize. Whether the thought comes from great literature or a bumper sticker, put it in your journal and assume that it will find its way into your life.

- At night, empty your day into your journal. Make note of what you learned and what you're thankful for. If you do a personal inventory in the evening, this can go into your journal, too.

The mechanics of keeping a journal aren't really important. You can buy very attractive, clothbound books with blank pages and write in those, but if you have a practical nature like I do, you'll prefer a

To Keep a Journal (*continued*)

. . . .

spiral notebook that stays flat and provides you with lines to write on. Be sure to write with a pen that feels good in your hand and glides easily across the paper: you can't "go with the flow" when your ballpoint is sticking. And don't fret about spelling or punctuation—your English teacher retired.

There's a lot to be said for keeping your journal in longhand, rather than using a computer. Nothing beats the mind-to-hand communication of writing with a pen on paper. Nevertheless, if you're more comfortable with a keyboard, journal there. Although most people choose to keep these private musings private, some swear by turning their journals into blogs so others can benefit. It's your call.

If, on the other hand, you're so private that you don't want to write down your innermost feelings and thoughts anywhere, remember that most of us either have lives that are much less interesting than we think or handwriting so poor that the curious wouldn't bother to decipher it. Unless you have special circumstances, your journal is probably quite safe in a drawer in your desk or nightstand. If you write something you'd rather no one ever sees, tear out the page and destroy it. It's yours to do with as you like.

You can save each journal you finish and go back to earlier ones as documentation of your ongoing growth. On days when you doubt your progress, old journals can be solid evidence of how far you've come. They're also testimonials to everything you've come through with the help of your Higher Power. You'll appreciate this resource when you're faced with difficulties that seem insurmountable.

So: if you can use a record of the past to enrich the present, keep your completed journals. Otherwise, clear away the space they take in your drawer and in your psyche. This is a new day. Write the date on top of the page. Claim it. It's yours.

none of us needs to become a contemplative cleric to benefit from prayer and meditation. Concentrated quiet time at some point during the day and remembering the spiritual foundation of our life and our recovery the rest of the time are sufficient for spawning miracles.

Saying grace at meals is especially appropriate for recovering food addicts. We can be thankful not only for having food to eat but for not abusing the food we have. If saying grace hasn't been a custom in your family, you may feel awkward about it at first. If that's the case, I suggest that you start to share a minute of silence before each meal. The people present can hold hands if they like. That minute may be used for a short prayer of gratitude, to remind yourself that the meal is in God's hands and you are, too. Those sixty seconds can also be a calming, centering time. Eating in this state of body and mind will make the food much more satisfying and it can even assist digestion.

Children are comfortable with graces and don't have nearly the inhibitions about them that some adults do. My daughter, when she was small, taught me some lovely ones. This one comes from the Waldorf schools founded by the late Austrian educator and Renaissance man Rudolf Steiner: "Earth who gives to us this food, Sun who makes it ripe and good, Dear Earth, Dear Sun, by you we live; our loving thanks to you we give." She adapted another from Robert Lewis Stevenson's *A Child's Garden of Verses*: "It is very nice to think the world is full of food and drink and little children saying grace in every sort of holy place." (I'm also fond of the impromptu grace that I overheard from a woman as she entered a buffet line: "OK, God, you're on.")

It also makes sense to have an after-meal prayer. When we binged, meals never stopped. A prayer can provide the parameters we need. A Protestant friend of mine attended a Catholic Mass and took note of the priest's closing words, "The Mass has ended. Go in peace." She turned that into an after-eating prayer: "The meal has ended. I go in peace."

Indeed, to go in peace is how we can best leave a meal, a meditation, or any other activity. The peace that comes from giving our food problem to a Higher Power and from practicing prayer and meditation comes to life when we express it. Remember that balance of our inner and outer lives? This is it: turning what we receive from going within into sharing, caring, giving, and growing in our world, our work, and our relationships.

Step 12 addresses this: "Having had a spiritual awakening as the result of these steps, we tried to carry this message to [others] and to practice these principles in all our affairs." Only this step includes the verb "to try." The others are quite clearly to be *done*, but because carrying the message implies a response from someone else, we can only give it our best shot.

More Revolutionary Concepts

. . . .

The Revolutionary Concepts introduced in Chapter Two had to do with you as a person and your relationship with food. The following ideas are revolutionary as well, but they pertain to you as a friend and partner and to your relationships with the people in your life. Read them every day this month.

- Recovery will touch every aspect of your life. You cannot change the way you relate to God, yourself, and food without also changing for the better the way you relate to other people.

- If you've tried to control your food and your weight, you've probably tried to control people, too.

- You have one life: your own. No one else's life belongs to you, not even your spouse's or your children's.

- You may truly believe that you know what other people should do, but that doesn't mean that they'll do it or even that it's your job to tell them. Just share your own experience.

- With the exception of extreme circumstances such as violence or abuse, no one makes you feel one way or another. You're the one who decides how you'll feel.

- Pleasing other people is fine as long as it pleases you, too. That doesn't mean that you should never be self-sacrificing. Just be sure that you want to do something for someone else before you do it, so you don't end up resenting it.

- You can listen compassionately to another person without feeling that you have to fix that person's life or situation.

- There's no better way to make a positive connection with another person than by being exactly who you are. You're the best *you* on record, and the genuine self of the other person will recognize your genuineness.

- The way to avoid having misunderstandings in relationships is to have no relationships. Having challenges in a relationship doesn't prove you a failure; it proves that you and the other person involved are human.

- Your opinions are as valid, your needs as important, and your life as precious as anyone else's. (This is true now, regardless of anything you've done, anything that's been done to you, how much you weigh, or what anyone says or thinks of you.)

- What other people think is not your concern. As long as you're true to yourself, let others think what they like. They will anyway.

More Revolutionary Concepts (*continued*)

. . . .

- Not every relationship is meant to last forever, and even those that last change.

- Having a relationship with food is much less difficult than having a relationship with a human being. The latter, however, is more rewarding and won't give you heartburn.

- Addictive people can have more than one addiction. An addictive relationship—one that's damaging but seemingly impossible to change or end—can impede your recovery. If you suspect that you need professional help or group support in this area, get it.

If you've taken advantage of the tremendous help that's available by contacting other recovering food addicts, you know that people who are putting these principles to work for themselves have turned theory into fact in a most impressive way. We need to be shown that spirituality isn't just Pollyanna pleasantness but that it can actually transport anyone who's willing and honest out of obsession, obesity, and despair to a life that's in order, a body that's healthy and comfortable, and an outlook that's hopeful—and with good reason. You can in turn offer this to others.

You don't need to wait until you're thin (that will eventually happen) or until you're perfect (that will never happen) to be of service to someone else. When I first began to look for a spiritual solution to binge eating, I was put in touch with a woman who proved to be very helpful. We had a wonderful long-distance conversation and just before our goodbyes she said, "Now call someone and give them whatever you've gotten from this talk."

"But I can't do that," I protested. "I just binged last night."

"There's somebody who binged this morning," she replied. "You have something they need."

I did what she told me. I called someone who I knew used food the way I did and let her know what I'd learned. Of course, I had to tell her that I was no expert and had binged only the night before. What I see now, though, is that no recovering addict is always an expert. Any of us could choose to go back to old ways of thought and action and be abusing food again in no time. Addicts who stay in recovery live in blessed moments, in the now, in a state of grace that keeps anxiety at bay. Because our new lives don't come from us as ego entities, we can only share with others in the company of good old humility.

Once your body is the way you want it, it's possible that you may want to forget where you came from. Years ago when I was still trying to control my eating with gimmicks and willpower, I lost weight through a commercial diet program and then got a job for the company. Everything went fine at first. But then I stopped relating to the people who came there for help. One day I unloaded to a coworker: "I am so sick of being around fat women!" It wasn't two weeks before I was back to binge eating and the start of a huge, rapid weight gain. At the time I hadn't a clue that I didn't want to deal with those "fat women" because I couldn't accept that I was one of them and would be all my life, regardless of what I weighed. I hadn't accepted my addiction, my vulnerability, or, to a great extent, my humanity. Going back to overeating was inevitable.

You can avoid such pitfalls by remembering love as your power source. In a support group, you'll have ample opportunities to share, but life itself offers such chances, too. People will ask how you lost weight, or they'll comment on how much happier or calmer you seem. When they do, tell them a little. If they're interested, they'll ask for more. The idea is to offer what you have without force-feeding anyone. It's possible for your enthusiasm to come across as fanatical zeal, leaving the impression that you've seen the light and are ready to outfit everybody else with the sunglasses they're sure to need shortly. It's important to tone that down. When you're established in recovery, you won't be out to make converts or reach a quota, but simply to be a resource about what made the difference for you.

One way to avoid being pushy is to speak with "I" messages instead of "you" messages. An "I" message is saying, "I found that I needed a spiritual solution for my food problem" rather than, "If you'd get some spirituality into your life, you could stop overeating, too." You've heard the old adage, "Your actions speak so loudly I can't hear the words you say." It's true. Our actions are chattering all the time, sometimes in shouts, sometimes in whispers, but they're always heard. When you've had a spiritual awakening, your life itself will carry the message—not just to other food addicts but to everyone you contact.

Hungry for Harmony

People are hungry for greater harmony, peace, and understanding. Without these, some overeat, some over-drink, some over-worry. Others stay moderate in their habits but never achieve more than moderate happiness. For people like these, just being in the same room with you once you've achieved inner peace could change their day. Being your friend could change their destiny. That's because *dis-ease* isn't the only thing that can be contagious. *Ease* can be contagious, too. In the same way that looking to others to be role models and confidantes is invaluable in your recovery, being those for other people will give your recovery strength and longevity.

It's that strong, day-by-day recovery that makes it possible to practice these principles in all our affairs. These principles will be obvious in your total way of living (for more on these principles, see Chapter Nine). Right now, though, while we're thinking about reaching out to others, let's consider how to incorporate these new ideals into personal relationships. It begins with the inventory steps and making amends. As your recovery progresses, you'll find yourself attracted to healthier relationships just as you'll be attracted to healthier foods.

As you continue with persistence and the willingness to let your Higher Power work in every area of your life, you'll find yourself living what at first seems to be a paradox. You'll love people more, but you'll be less attached. You'll be able to let go emotionally, freeing the people you care about to be themselves—their best selves. You'll stop trying to control other people in the same way you've stopped trying to control your food and your weight. You'll accept people precisely as they are because you accept yourself precisely as you are.

There are plenty of good books available on improving relationships, and you may find them helpful in learning techniques for better communication and for relating more confidently to others. Strictly by virtue of what's taking place within you as you overcome your addiction, however, you can expect your dealings with those around you to improve. If they don't, you'll be equipped to take positive ac-

Striking a Balance

. . . .

Keeping your recovery strong and viable depends on two responsibilities: continued surrender of your eating problem to a Higher Power, and maintaining the balance of a healthy spiritual life and a healthy life, spiritually lived. The following suggestions may help you come to this balance of "looking in, reaching out."

Make personal inventory an ongoing practice. Be on the lookout—and I'm paraphrasing the book *Alcoholics Anonymous* here—for selfishness, dishonesty, resentment, and fear. When you see these, let your Higher Power take them; discuss them with another person, make apologies or take other action if indicated; and set your mind on helping others.

Review your day before you go to sleep. Is there something you want to talk about with God or another person? Is there some situation left from today that you want to take care of tomorrow? What progress have you seen in yourself today? What is there in your day that pleases you or that you can be proud of? Thank your Higher Power, and give yourself some credit, too. You're doing great.

Pray and meditate every day. Take some quiet time for yourself. Prayer and meditation are simply an expansion of that. Use your quiet time to read something soothing or inspiring, write in your journal, read or say any prayers that are meaningful to you, talk with God, or tend to the specific devotions that may be part of your religious faith. Spend some of this time in silent meditation, using the breath-counting technique or another method to still your mind and be open to your Higher Power.

Share what you've found with others. Sharing is offering, not forcing. As you recover, you'll find ways to share nonintrusively and beneficially, particularly if you're part of a support group. Remember, too, that your life itself carries a message to other food addicts and to everyone around you.

Remember your new way of life in all your activities and relationships. As someone relying on spiritual truths to recover from food obsession, you'll be living a spiritual life. This doesn't imply prudish piety. It does, however, call for putting all of your actions and your dealings with people on a spiritual basis. As you live this new way and make contact with your Higher Power in prayer and meditation, much of this will come to you intuitively. You'll look for something of God in everyone around you. You'll allow other people to be who they are. You'll be able to accept others as they are and—especially—accept yourself as you are.

tion. Unhealthy relationships that you may have tolerated before your love-empowerment began will be like the clothes you wore then: they'll require some alterations.

Be patient with those who are watching you change. Remember that another's transformation can be threatening. Those you love need to know that you're not abandoning them as you become more fully who you really are. On the other hand, never allow someone else's fear of your growth to impede it. Your primary obligation is to your own unfolding. When you're committed to that, your commitment to your family, friends, and colleagues will have the best possible foundation.

Looking within for guidance and reaching out to get and give more of the same will make you a better friend and a better partner—not just to other people in your life but to yourself as well. You'll treat others with fairness and respect, and you'll accept no less from them. You'll be learning to love in the truest sense of the word because you'll be learning from love itself. This is part of how the process works, part of the way your thinking/feeling nature must work if you are to live addiction-free. If you came to this way of life only hoping to lose weight, this is one remarkable bonus.

CHAPTER FIVE

THE GIFT OF CHOICE

You've embarked upon an inner journey. Its destination—spiritual awakening—is not like a port or station. You won't arrive, unpack your bags, and be done with it. It is instead opening a door to a new way of life, one lived on a daily basis, renewable every morning. And every morning a spiritual gift will be waiting for you, just as surely as if it were a wrapped package with your name on the tag. That's the gift of choice.

There's no choice when eating for a fix. We did it when we thought that we wanted to and when we knew that we didn't, yet the idea of refraining from it was paralyzing because we thought that it meant our choice would be taken away. In truth, however, it's only when we're set free from having to overeat or undereat, reward ourselves with food or punish ourselves with deprivation, that we really have a choice at all. Only then can we make choices about our lives—to treat ourselves well, for example—and about our food.

As a recovering food addict, you'll need to learn how to use the gift of choice the same way you've learned to use tangible gifts, from your first bike to your new computer. In the throes of the addiction, many choices were limited. You wore an outfit because it was one that fit. Perhaps you took a certain job because you didn't feel good enough about yourself to apply for the other one—the one you really wanted. And if you're like me, you certainly ate one particular food or another not because you really wanted it or even because it tasted all that great, but because it was around or it was the one that offered the kick (or the sedation) you needed at the time.

In recovery, choices abound. With a reprieve from food obsession and a commitment to love-powered rather than ego-powered living, you'll be able to:

- Believe that you're OK because "God doesn't make junk"
- Experience compassion
- Express your feelings
- Accept life instead of fighting it
- Have fun
- Welcome supportive friends
- Go into your world with love instead of fear
- Feel good physically and emotionally
- Give to life and enjoy the rewards of giving
- Ease up on yourself
- Forgive yourself and others
- Reach out to people
- Take risks
- Look on the bright side
- Find humor in almost every situation
- Rejoice in others' good fortune as well as your own
- Take good care of yourself
- Be grateful
- Delight in the little things
- Feel attractive
- Be honest
- Smile
- Look forward to every day
- Unleash your creativity
- Grow
- Learn from difficulties

- See the beauty around you
- Put more beauty around you
- Love
- Be happy

Can you see that all these are choices? Does it make sense to you that we can choose, for example, to be happy, or does it seem that happiness has to happen to us, that it's the result of a hefty raise, a smart purchase, or a fresh compliment? Of course, these things give us a boost. It's wonderful when they happen. That boost, however, is not happiness. Happiness is far less flighty. It comes from within and depends on little else. It's a choice. This doesn't mean that there will never be challenges, dilemmas, problems, and losses, even major ones. Feeling frustration, anger, and grief regarding these is natural, but your underlying sense of wellbeing—real happiness—will still be with you if you choose to have it.

There certainly may be times when you'll choose to feel unhappy. That's all right. You may want to give yourself an unhappiness allotment of an hour or two, and then get on with whatever it takes to put you back in touch with the reality that you can indeed choose to be happy. "Whatever it takes" will probably be one of the same methods you're already using to postpone inappropriate eating: talking with another person, getting a change of scenery, or having a quiet time for prayer, journal writing, or meditation. Do whatever you need to do.

It isn't always easy to remember that you're choosing your own feelings, but you can go on the *premise* that all these choices are yours, and you'll soon see that the premise is correct. The ability to make choices is a gift from life to you. There are two choices, however, that recovering food addicts need to make each day: (1) to remember that our lives are now in the care of a Higher Power, and (2) to refrain from eating for a fix.

As for the first of these choices, if you're working through the Twelve Steps, you made a decision to allow your Higher Power to take care of your will and your life back at Step 3. That decision was like deciding to take a job. Choosing each day to remember the decision is like showing up for work at nine AM prepared to do the best you can.

The Now Choice

. . . .

We can accept the gift of choice only in the present moment. Certainly our lives are enriched by happy memories and fond hopes. We can learn from the past and we must plan for the future, but we're asking for trouble when we try to live in either one. Focusing on the past invites regret and remorse. Denying the present for the future guarantees worry and anxiety. Why? Because neither the past nor the future is real. The only reality is this moment. Some people call this the eternal now.

We are thoroughly in the present when we are engrossed in a project and lose track of time. That's when we aren't judging ourselves, when we aren't too late or too early, too young or too old, when we're not concerned about what we've eaten or how much we weigh or anything else. We're in the process of being alive. In even a long life, the hours of being fully, blissfully alive can be few indeed. For many people, most in-the-now time is enjoyed during childhood. Children are grounded in the present to a degree that can be unnerving to adults.

In recovery, we can reclaim a degree of this childlikeness in allowing ourselves to be thoroughly in the present. Food addiction is often accompanied by an ongoing neglect of the present, replacing the attention that today deserves with a focus on last year's thinness or next week's diet. I'm partial to the line in the Lord's Prayer that says, "Give us this day our daily bread." This day. That's it. For years I was unwilling to gratefully accept my daily bread: I wanted several days' bread with honey and butter and cheese.

Living in the now is one way to come to know through and through that this day's bread—and time and inspiration and whatever else I need—is here for me today. For today, I'm taken care of. So are you.

Growth in recovery is a daily proposition. We can no more live on yesterday's spirituality than on yesterday's oxygen. We claim today's spirituality by making the now choice, by choosing to remember that:

(a) This is the only moment there is.

(b) This is the only moment we have access to our Higher Power.

(c) This is the only moment we can refrain from eating for a fix—and this is the only moment we need to.

When you operate from the supposition that your Higher Power (be it God, love, or the collective power of a group of recovering individuals) is handling the outcome of situations, you're free to take care of what's in front of you. Don't believe for a minute that this means resigning yourself to dullness, drudgery, and an uneventful life. When you team up with the power of love, what will be in front of you to do will oftentimes surpass your wildest dreams. Of course, there will be *some* dullness, drudgery, and uneventfulness. A full life comes in all colors, including a little gray.

You implement the second daily choice, to refrain from eating for a fix, every time you use Chapter Three's suggested postponement techniques and every time you elect to sit with your feelings without anything to eat, drink, or chew. Therefore, you're already aware that choosing to refrain from eating for a fix bears little resemblance to going on a willpower diet. Dieting can, in fact, impede your progress because it gives the illusion that you're controlling your eating, which, for any true food addict, is a dangerous fallacy. What is required in terms of food choices is a new way of eating that arises from this new way of thinking.

As your recovery proceeds, refraining from eating for a fix won't even seem like making a choice. It will be a non-issue, in the same category as having to choose between buying a jet or a small island in the Caribbean. That degree of freedom is incredible for those of us who've had difficulty getting through just one hour without obsessing over food. Nevertheless, eating for a fix can be virtually guaranteed to any food addict who goes back to former patterns of thought and action. Therefore, whenever you keep harmful or unnecessary food out of your mouth—even if this requires no conscious effort because you simply don't want it—you've already made the choice to refrain from eating for a fix. You're unconsciously acting on that choice and your appetite itself has responded to the choice you've made.

I call these times "state-of-grace days" because we don't have to earn them. We only have to accept them. Expect to enjoy ever greater numbers of these as time goes by. On some days, though—and in the beginning it may be *all* days—you'll still want to eat the way you always have. This isn't terrible and it doesn't mean that you're a failure.

Your cravings may spring from something missing in your spiritual life. Use this opportunity to look at your recovery practices:

- Do you recognize that your own power is useless when it comes to food?
- Are you looking to your Higher Power for help?
- Are you willing to postpone the fix and sit with your feelings?
- Do you need to let go of some shame or guilt or resentment that hasn't been dealt with?
- Would it help to talk things over with someone?
- Do you owe amends?
- Have you been taking time for prayer and meditation?
- Are you sharing with others?
- Are you using spiritual principles in all aspects of your life, those that have to do with your eating and those that don't?

Sometimes taking a single action to deepen your spiritual life can rid you of the most stubborn food craving. If you can't pinpoint exactly what's amiss, just do something. Take a half-hour for journal writing and meditating, or call someone you know who's having a difficult time and offer that person a patient ear.

Perhaps your desire to overeat has a physical basis. Maybe you really are hungry—have you been eating enough? Or you may have recently eaten a particular food that, for you, incited an obsessive pattern.

Another possibility is that there may be a lack of balance in your physical/emotional self. Could you be expecting too much of yourself? To give a personal example, I like having lunch by myself. It's not all the time—that much isolation with food would tell me I was headed for trouble—but when I'm not slated to dine in company, I look forward to that midday hiatus to read, regroup, and have a silent meal alone.

Now, my husband and I both work at home. He usually goes out on his own to eat and read the daily papers, but when he unexpectedly decides to stay around and I've been looking forward to that alone time, I really have to take care of myself. If I can take five minutes of quiet and center myself and come to appreciate the chance to spend time with him, that's great. If I can't get there, I find that accepting I need lunch alone is smarter than trying to be flexible. I'm a compulsive overeater. Even in recovery, there's sometimes a limit to my flexibility.

The anonymous programs use the acronym HALT to remind their members not to get too hungry, too angry, too lonely, or too tired. When you want to extend a meal beyond reasonable parameters or eat what you know is extra, unnecessary food between meals, examine your life in terms of HALT. You may have two or three of the danger signals operating without realizing it. Take care of them. This is another reason to stay away from diets. On most of them, you're hungry from lack of food, angry about being on a diet, lonely because so much socializing takes place around food, and tired from lack of nutrients or from trying to restrain yourself.

On those hungry days, you'll need to make the conscious choice to refrain from eating for a fix—and you may need to do it more than once. The difference between choosing to abstain from damaging eating and using willpower to stick to a diet is surrender versus combat. The struggle ends when you surrender the inclination, desire, or compulsion to misuse food to the power of love.

A Willow's Flexibility

You can surrender perfectionism at the same time you surrender your compulsion to misuse food. When you're no longer eating for a fix, you'll still sometimes eat more than you need. You might make a food choice that you wish afterward had been different. When these things happen, you won't have "broken your diet," because there's no diet to break. You'll have a willow's flexibility to withstand storms that would demolish an oak. Without having to reach some nebulous state of perfection, either in your life or at your meals, you'll be living out your choice to be free of the food fix one day after the next.

Another choice that will be yours in recovery is that of choosing what you'll eat. You don't simply "stop and stay stopped" as you might with another addiction. You need to stop abusing food but still decide what to prepare or what to order for breakfast, lunch, and dinner. Knowing what to eat and how much can be scary. After all, food seems to have been the cause of so much misery. How do you know that you can trust it or that you can trust yourself to make decisions about it?

You may remember the times when you fasted or went on liquid diets, only to find your peacefulness broken when you had to return to eating solid food. Part of

Actions that Change Attitudes toward Food

. . . .

1. Allow an inner transformation to take place through bringing your spiritual life to bear on your life as a whole— eating included. Using the Twelve Steps is one proven way to do this.

2. Find at least one person, preferably a group of people, with whom you can talk about your attitudes toward food whenever you need to. As soon as you're able, provide the same sort of support for others.

3. Bring your Higher Power into food situations with you. You aren't alone when you remember that the God of your understanding is with you all the time. This help is not only available in dramatic situations but at banquets, buffets, and when passing a bakery window.

4. Be grateful for your food. Say a prayer of thanks at meals. Remember the contribution of everyone and every-thing, from the earthworms to the farmers, the retailer to the cook (even if that's you).

5. Choose beautiful foods and present them beautifully. Your tongue may prefer ice cream to strawberries, but your eyes are partial to strawberries. Indulge them for a change. Experience your meals with all your senses. Eat slowly. Put flowers on the table and play soft music—not just for company, for you, too.

6. Select and prepare your foods with care, even reverence. Think about what it means to serve food to yourself and others. You're providing physical sustenance that will become a part of your living body and the bodies of people you care about. You deserve the best and so do they. This is a sacred trust.

7. Discover the clean delight of simple food. I remember the first time I had a cup of tea without lemon or milk or sweetener. I was amazed at how delicately flavorful it was, how inter-esting to taste something I'd drunk so often before without really experienc-ing it. You can discover something similar with an unbuttered potato, a ripe peach, or a simple salad of farm-fresh greens. Food certainly doesn't have to be bland or dull, but it's curious that for people who suppos-edly love food, we don't actually know what most of it tastes like.

8. Learn to feel safe between meals. Sit with the feeling of not being full, the way you've learned to sit with other feelings. Don't get Spartan about it (that's a dieter's mentality or even the anorexic's), but get to know how it

Actions that Change Attitudes toward Food (*continued*)

. . . .

feels to get a break from digesting food. Realize that you can be content without being full.

9. Conversely, experience fullness. It's easy to ignore the body's signals that say "enough." Some people think that the bodies of chronic overeaters don't even produce these signals anymore, but I believe we've simply ignored them. Pay attention. How does it feel to be full? Can you accept the truth that you're safe after a meal and you're safe before one? It's all right to have a full stomach or an empty stomach. All humans and nonhuman animals at times have one, at times the other. Join the biosphere!

10. Explore the world around you. Thinking about eating and thinking about not eating have taken up enough valuable time. It's a wonderland out there! What do you really want to do? Would you like to take acting lessons, learn to knit, play golf, work for a cause, speak Italian, write short stories? Do it—not after you've had something to eat and not after you lose ten pounds. Do it now.

the appeal of such programs is that with them you don't need to have anything to do with food—out of sight, out of mind. But just as you can't learn to swim on dry land, you can't learn to eat in a loving way, or even come to know that it's possible, until you try it.

The Freedom to Choose

The inner change you're offered will render you capable of dealing with life as it is. Part of this life—for human beings and every other animal on the planet—is to eat. Although any addict who expects to get well must respect the severity of addiction, fear doesn't heal anybody. Love does the healing, and love and fear cannot work in the same space. If you're afraid of food, put that on the fear list in your personal inventory and ask your Higher Power take the fear away. You can expect to develop a new, respectful, but fearless attitude toward food.

If you started turning to food when you were a child, you evidently needed it to shield you from things you feared or didn't understand. Some people with eating disorders were physically, mentally, or sexually abused as children; but even in happy homes, some needs go unmet. Then, the food was a friend, a helper, a protector. It can't help you anymore and you don't need its brand of protection, but it can become a friend in a sane, mature way—the way you may now admire and enjoy a sibling whom you envied or resented as a child. Your attitude has changed. Your attitude toward food can change as well.

As your attitude changes, you'll make food choices from a different vantage point. When, for example, you were eating for emotional solace, you may have gravitated toward sweet, creamy foods that were nutritionally marginal. With a different motivation for eating—the desire to nourish yourself for the healthiest, happiest life possible—you're a ripe candidate for an attitude adjustment. You will, in effect, be making a shift: Food will no longer get star status, either as hero or villain. It will instead play an important but low-key supporting role.

You're in the ideal place for allowing your attitudes toward food to change because you've been working from the inside out: looking at yourself first, then at your food. Dr. Dean Ornish, author of *Eat More, Weigh Less*, used this approach with his heart patients, many of whom were overweight, in his groundbreaking work that showed that cardiovascular disease could be reversed through a program that includes yoga and meditation, group support, moderate exercise, and a low-fat vegetarian diet. He explains the role of inner change in this way: "It's not enough to simply change behaviors without dealing with deeper issues. Telling someone who's lonely and depressed and isolated that by changing her diet, she'll live longer isn't very motivating. Who wants to live longer if they feel bad? So we address the emotional and spiritual dimensions of health and illness, not just the physical. When you feel happier and more peaceful, you tend to choose behaviors that are life-enhancing, rather than self-destructive."

One life-enhancing behavior is to choose life-enhancing foods. Think about this concept for a minute. Life-enhancing foods should look good, smell good, and be appealing in their own right. Just because some food is low-calorie, low-fat, low-carb, or supposedly good for you doesn't necessarily qualify it as life-enhancing. Do you have any childhood memories of having to eat liver or cooked spinach or something else you detested? You may have swallowed it and ingested some nutrients in the process, but it's doubtful that you felt your life had been enhanced.

My friend Suzanne is an inspiration when it comes to life-enhancing food. After she changed her attitudes through spiritual principles, she set about changing her food attitudes most decisively. She cleaned out her kitchen and got rid of everything that didn't add to the health of her body or the beauty of her cupboards. Most of the packaged snack foods went, along with the white sugar and bleached flour. She filled her shelves with tawny grains and colorful beans stored in handsome apothecary jars she found at a yard sale. Fresh fruit was always ripening on her table or counter, and after she befriended an organic gardener, she learned to grow sprouts and dry apples (and to notice sunrises, sunsets, and the phases of the moon). She started making juices from concord grapes and Rome Beauty apples and concocting colorful smoothies for breakfast. My friend who had already been beautiful to those who knew her became strikingly so to everyone she met. Her eyes looked bluer than they had been before. Her skin seemed translucent. Her body responded to this treatment with glowing health and increased energy.

We influence each other more than we know. Whenever I'm tempted to throw something together instead of lovingly prepare fresh food, I think of Suzanne. Then the need to rush abates a bit. I put away the can opener and get out the paring knife.

There is no single, rigid way to eat that's right for everyone. We have different activity levels and different ethnic backgrounds. We live in different climates and in different social environments. Nevertheless, physiologically we are quite similar. Based on that similarity, there are guidelines about eating that apply to humans as a species. It makes sense, for instance, to eat primarily foods that come to us from nature rather than expecting the body to deal with synthetic substances it doesn't understand.

It's known, too, that a diet high in animal fat, other saturated fats, and artificial trans fats, is the foremost contributor to heart disease—the number one killer in this country. It's also been linked to several kinds of cancer, Type II diabetes, osteoporosis, and many other plagues of civilization, being overweight in-

Before You Choose Your Foods

. . . .

Before you choose your foods, make this choice: *choose to love yourself with the food you eat.* Many food addicts say, "When I was growing up, food meant love in my house," and they use that to rationalize overeating today. There's a hole in that reasoning, though. Maybe love was expressed to you as a child through food, but if you're abusing food now, you're abusing yourself. That's not love.

Decide to love yourself with how you eat just as you're learning to love yourself with how you live. Some of the following suggestions will seem familiar. You may have even tried them. What's different this time, however, is that you're now engaged in a transformational process that's spiritual and thereby total. That transformation will make it possible for you to implement these suggestions, even if you've tried them and failed in the past. In fact, as your inner transformation continues, you'll see that you will be taking many of these measures without giving them any thought. You'll read this list and say, "Hey, I'm doing that."

- **Eat without guilt.** Guilt enjoys its own company. The guiltier you feel, the more likely you are to continue the guilt-producing behavior. Affirm: *I eat in love, not in guilt.*

- **Eat for your health.** Don't pass this one by because it seems so obvious. How many people do you know who truly choose their foods to bring about high-level health? Precious few. Be one of them. *Affirm: I eat for high-level health.*

- **Eat slowly.** Even if you have only a half-hour lunch break, don't inhale your food. Chew it. Taste it. If meals are routinely rushed or interrupted (if you work on call or if you're the parent of small children), make a point of slowing down and sitting down for at least one leisurely meal each day. *Affirm: I eat slowly. There's plenty of time.*

- **Eat when you're calm and centered.** If you're upset, don't eat, even if it's mealtime. Pray. Take a walk or a bath. Phone someone. Sane eating and inner turmoil are rarely found at the same table. *Affirm: I eat only when I am calm and centered. Or: I give myself the gift of becoming centered before every meal.*

- **Eat the way that's best for you, regardless of others' opinions.** The majority of people are far superior to the food they eat. Every human being is a divine creation entitled to the very best, yet most people in our culture eat quantities of fast, fragmented,

Before You Choose Your Foods (*continued*)

. . . .

and "foodless" food. When you stop joining them in this, they're liable to rib you about being a health nut or a goody-goody. You're neither; continue to do what's right for you. *Affirm: I eat in the way that is best for me, regardless of anyone else's opinion.*

- **Eat food prepared with love, care, and attention.** When you're the chef, prepare your food in this way. When you eat out, choose places where you're most likely to get food that has had love, care, and attention given it. Many restaurant proprietors are as concerned with these intangibles as with the special of the day—and not just at expensive restaurants either. Look for those that feature fresh foods, that are privately owned and have the owner on the premises, and that specialize in natural foods. In many cases, an ethnic restaurant, particularly if it's family owned, is a good place to dine. *Affirm: I eat only food prepared with love, care, and attention. Or I prepare this food with love, care, and attention.*

- **Allow your tastes and preferences to change for the better.** When you're committed to treating yourself well with the foods you eat, you're willing to make some changes, try some new things. You probably won't like all of them and you don't need to, but you can allow your tastes and preferences to change so you come to appreciate new textures, subtle flavors, and lighter versions of favorite dishes. *Affirm: I allow my tastes and preferences to change for the better.*

- **Let your food choices express who you are.** You're a beautiful, healthy, compassionate, intelligent human being. Select foods that are beautiful to look at, smell, and taste; that contribute to your health; that express compassion to others; and that are the result of intelligent discernment. *Affirm: I let my food choices express who I am. Or, I make food choices that express beauty, healthfulness, intelligence, and compassion.*

cluded. People who choose natural foods that are low in fat are healthier, as a rule, than those who eat processed and high-fat foods. Their bodies are leaner, although they eat heartily. In parts of the world where this style of eating is the norm, obesity is virtually unknown. Recovering food addicts who eat in this way don't have to be so concerned about their weight, portion sizes, or cutting back after weekends or holidays.

Combining a spiritual turnaround and this gentle way of eating brings this loving approach full circle. Spirituality is the inner side; gentle, natural food choices the outer. Those who make natural food choices find that these support and complement their total way of living. It may well be that a new way of life deserves—and perhaps demands—a new way of eating. Your spiritual awakening provides you with the gift of choice. All you have to do is unwrap it.

CHAPTER SIX

THE LOVE-POWERED DIET

Most people who have battled food have done exactly that: battled. But with the principles you've been incorporating into your thinking and living, the kitchen no longer needs to be a war zone. We've discussed the spiritual and emotional aspects of this new way of life first so that your food choices can now reflect those spiritual and emotional changes.

We're about to explore a lifesaving and life-affirming way of eating that I believe mirrors spiritual growth and emotional stability. It's a way of eating that study after study has shown to "do your body good," and it sends feelings of deprivation packing. Expecting any foodstyle to cure a food addict would be like expecting a drug to cure a drug addict. It will take more than an eating plan, however enlightened, to heal the emotional wounds that you may have tried to salve with food. Therefore, it's critical that you learn to live in conscious contact with the love that's able to give you the emotional strength that no food can provide. Allowing yourself to be reshaped from the inside out forms the foundation.

At this point, you're ready to tap the power of love to help you make food choices that will not only help you get your weight where you want it, but will uplift you emotionally and spiritually. It's important to realize that when that power of love touches you anywhere, it touches you everywhere. In this case, wanting to have it all—peace with food, peace with your body, peace within—isn't greed; it's good sense.

So, what does love have to do with the way you eat? Chances are, it hasn't had much to do with it, and that's what put you in the pickle that led you to this book. But surely no loving God and no loving part of yourself wants you tormented by food cravings, subject to depressing and even dangerous diets, or risking your life with morbid obesity or a binge/purge merry-go-round that ceases to be merry long before the ride is over. It also stands to reason that a loving God or your most loving self would be interested in your overall welfare and the welfare of all people, all forms of life, and an Earth so nurturing we easily call her *mother*.

Because love encompasses everything, nothing is unimportant, including tonight's dinner menu. Think about it for a minute. If you were pure love, the loving parent of all life, how would you want people to eat? I think it would be a way that:

- Is generous, delicious, and aesthetically pleasing
- Promotes high-level health as well as normal weight
- Is economical and provides plenty for everybody
- Respects all life, and
- Is environmentally sustainable

That describes a love-powered diet.

Diet can be an ugly word, and sentences like "I'm a fat slob and ought to go on a diet" or "I was bad and blew my diet" are no less than obscene. I'm using the word differently here. The love-powered diet applies to a natural, gentle style of eating that uses the d-word in its general and non-threatening sense, as when you say, "I make sure that my children get a good diet." What people eat is their *diet*. Depriving oneself in order to lose weight is *dieting*. What we're talking about is a way of eating that uses love's power instead of willpower to make change stick.

There's no dieting here—no menus, no amounts, no absolutes. Why should I tell you what to eat on some hypothetical days one through seven as if you had only a week to live? You have a life to live, and it isn't hypothetical. Besides, in real life every day is "day one." At this point in your progress along the continuum of inner to outer wellbeing, you're ready for recommendations, not regimentation. You don't need rules to resist but tools to get new concepts off the drawing board and into practice.

The love-powered diet celebrates the abundance of nature. Its basic food groups are:

- Fruits, preferably fresh but also frozen, unsweetened
- Vegetables (salads, crudités, and steamed, sautéed, and baked veggies, with an emphasis on super-nutritious leafy greens); the starchy vegetables including potatoes, yams, and corn belong here nutritionally as well, although in terms of meal-planning, you'll often be using them the way you'd use grains
- Whole grains, including whole wheat (bread, bulghur, pasta, etc.), brown rice, oats, cornmeal (cornbread, polenta), buckwheat (pancakes, noodles), and gourmet grains such as millet, quinoa, and amaranth
- Legumes, such as dried beans (navy, kidney, red, pink, lima, garbanzo), peas, lentils, and soybeans (i.e., edamame) and soy foods such as tofu and tempeh

There's also an auxiliary category of rich foods that are higher in oil content or in natural sugars than the basic foods. They are used in smaller quantities as condiments or garnishes and can supplement the diet of people who need extra calories to maintain their weight. "Rich relatives" include nuts and seeds (preferably raw and unsalted), olives, avocado, extra-virgin olive oil; dried fruits, fruit juices, all-fruit jam; and sweeteners such as agave nectar, sorghum, and pure maple syrup.

This translates into meals such as fruit plates and fruit smoothies; crisp salads and vegetable stir-fries; casseroles and chowders; sandwiches on hearty whole-wheat bread and quick loaves like cornbread and banana bread served with served with satisfying soups such as lentil and split pea; an assortment of rice and noodle dishes; beans and rice, beans on toast, and Boston baked beans; veggie-burgers, veggie wraps, or a breakfast-style supper of scrambled tofu, grilled onions and tomatoes, and vegetarian Canadian "bacon" in the refrigerator section of any natural food store. The world of ethnic cooking comes alive for love-powered chefs, too. You can experiment with dishes from:

- The Middle East: pita sandwiches with hummus (chickpea spread) or baba ghannouj (eggplant dip), tabbouleh (cracked-wheat salad), rice pilafs
- Italy: eggplant dishes, gnocchi, and an endless array of pasta with vegetables and tomato or wine-based sauces
- India: a variety of vegetable curries with tantalizing complementary chutneys, dal (spicy sauces made from lentils or split peas), pungent rice dishes
- Mexico: chili sans carne, avocado tostadas, bean burritos, vegetable fajitas
- Asia: vegetable sushi with miso soup and seaweed salad at the Japanese place; steamed veggies and brown rice with garlic sauce on the side from the Chinese delivery guy; the potato, cabbage, and tofu dish from the Vietnamese restaurant; and the cellophane noodles with lotus root and exotic vegetables from the Thai café

Even in traditional American fare you can make easy shifts, such as a veggie-burger for hamburger. You can customize what you eat to the way you live.

This may all sound a little fishy (or not fishy enough) because you've figured out that I'm talking about a plant-based diet or, to call it what it is, a vegetarian diet—vegan, even, meaning that, if you do this completely, you'll be creating your meals with no products of animal origin. Let me reassure you that eating solely from the plant kingdom—most of the time or even all of the time— need not change your politics, your religion, or any other part of yourself that the label *vegetarian* or *vegan* doesn't seem to fit. You never need to use these words if you're not comfortable with them. Some prominent proponents of this way of eating, such as Caldwell Esselstyn, M.D., author of *Prevent and Reverse Heart Disease*, don't use them at all. And because the love-powered diet doesn't require absolute adherence, you can start to make progress even before you've gone "all the way."

Some people read about the horrors of factory farming and the slaughter industry, and become vegans overnight. Others might follow a scenario like this:

- They stop eating land animals first (cows, pigs, chickens)
- Then eggs (factory-farmed eggs are a product of intense cruelty, and because there's little oversight on so-called free-range eggs, it's easier to simply let them go)

- Then aquatic animals (fish)
- Then dairy products (milk and cheese)

Other people cut out dairy first, and find that once they've made the break from their cheese/pizza/ice cream/yogurt addiction, everything else is easy. (*Don't Drink Your Milk* by Frank Oski, M.D., is a real eye-opener.) The way you get to where you're going isn't nearly as important as that you leave where you are.

Read the list (opposite) of famous vegetarians of the past and present; you'll soon discover that if you do decide to join them, you'll be in good company.

A Taste for Quality

Love-powered dining doesn't just bypass animal foods. It also gives short shrift to the highly refined, overly processed, phony foods that we're fond of calling junk.

Although we're making progress and real food is showing up where it never did before, the majority of items found in convenience stores and gas stations, much of what's in an ordinary bakery, and just about all the offerings at the movie theater are still likely to be junk food. The supermarket has its share of nutritionally vacant items, and some of them even creep into health food stores. Reading labels is a good practice, but the best food is fresh food—fruits and vegetables from the orchard and garden that have no packaging and no label.

For a love-powered diet to give you all it can, you'll want to avoid any food that isn't good enough for you—just the way your mother may have told you not to date a particular boy (or girl) for that very reason. If it's high in sugar (when sugar is near the top of an ingredients list, it's high), high in salt (enough to make you thirsty), or very fatty (if it's fried, "melts in your mouth," or leaves a shine on your napkin), it's not up to your standards.

Everyone knows that junk food is a nutritional disaster, packs in the calories, and causes a yen for more of the same. In addition, it simply isn't becoming to people who are out to love themselves more. You can go to an elegant restaurant and consume a thousand calories in a special dinner with a special person and leave feeling terrific about the world and everything that's in it, yourself included. Or you can

Some Famous Vegetarians, Past and Present

. . . .

Philosophy and Religion

Buddha
Clement of Alexandria
Ralph Waldo Emerson
J. Krishnamurti
Plato
Pythagoras
Jean-Jacques Rousseau
Socrates
Henry David Thoreau
John Wesley
Ellen G. White

Literature and Journalism

Louisa May Alcott
Franz Kafka
John Milton
Malcolm Muggeridge
George Bernard Shaw
Percy Bysshe Shelley
Upton Sinclair
Isaac Bashevis Singer
Sir Rabindranath Tagore
Leo Tolstoy
Alice Walker

Science and Medicine

Max Bircher-Benner
Deepak Chopra
Charles Darwin
Thomas Edison
Albert Einstein

Sylvester Graham
John Harvey Kellogg
Sir Isaac Newton
Albert Schweitzer
Benjamin Spock
Leonardo da Vinci

Politcs and Social Reform

Susan B. Anthony
Clara Barton
Annie Besant
General William Booth
Julio Cesar Chavez
Mahatma Gandhi
Horace Greeley
Henry Heimlich
Dennis Kucinich
Helen and Scott Nearing
Gloria Steinem
John Wesley

Sports

Hank Aaron
    (baseball legend)
Ridgely Abele (World
    Championship, karate)
Andeas Cahling (Mr. Inter-
    national, bodybuilding)
Bill Goldberg (World
    Champion pro-wrestler)
Ruth Heidrich
    (Ironman triathlete)

Desmond Howard (NFL)
Jim Kaat (Hall of Fame
    pitcher)
Billie Jean King
    (tennis champion)
Killer Kowalski (wrestler)
Tony LaRussa (manager,
    St. Louis Cardinals
    baseball team)
Mark Levey
    (Buffalo Bills coach)
Sixto Linares (world
    record holder, twenty-
    four-hour triathlon)
Edwin Moses
    (Olympic gold
    medalist, undefeated
    for eight years in
    400-meter hurdles)
Martina Navratilova
    (tennis great)
Bill Pearl (four-time
    Mr. Universe)
Bill Pickering (World
    Record, swimming
    the English Channel)
Bill Player (golfer)
Stan Price (world record,
    bench press)
Murray Rose (world
    records for both
    400- and 1500- meter
    freestyle, swimming)

Some Famous Vegetarians, Past and Present (Continued)

. . . .

Entertainment

Casey Affleck	Dre (Outkast)	Morrissey
Fiona Apple	Melissa Etheridge	Olivia Newton-John
India Arie	Dick Gregory	Stevie Nicks
Rosanna Arquette	Josh Hartnett	Anna Paquin
Erykah Badu	Woody Harrelson	Joaquin Phoenix
Bob Barker	Anne Hathaway	Natalie Portman
Drew Barrymore	Dustin Hoffman	Phylicia Rashad
Angela Bassett	Lisa Kudrow	Ravi Shankar
Jeff Beck	k.d. Lang	Alicia Silverstone
Ed Begley, Jr.	Avril Lavigne	Russell Simmons
Orlando Bloom	Cloris Leachman	Shania Twain
Lisa Bonet	Annie Lennox	Carrie Underwood
Brandy	Benji Madden (Good	Lindsay Wagner
Ellen Burstyn	Charlotte)	Forest Whitaker
Julie Christie	Alyssa Milano	Vanessa Williams
Emily Deschanel	Moby	Paul Winter
	Sir Paul McCartney	
	Mary Tyler Moore	

go to some fast-food place, gobble up a thousand calories in 4.2 minutes, and feel fat and guilty as you toss the wrappers. Cultivate your taste for quality food and select the best food that you can afford.

Go for quality drinks, too, since many are questionable. Alcohol, with its empty calories and mood-altering potential, should be limited to moderate consumption, if you choose to drink at all. A typical soda contains some nine teaspoons of sugar in a twelve-ounce can, and no artificial sweetener has been proven unequivocally safe.

The caffeine in cola as well as in coffee and black tea can also be a problem. Caffeine is a stimulant. The easiest way to modify a caffeine-induced buzz is to eat, and many people do this unconsciously. Caffeine can also suppress the appetite temporarily, but it comes back like gangbusters. Dieters usually drink lots of coffee, tea, and cola, and dieters usually relapse. It's possible that there is a caffeine connection.

According to Agatha Thrash, M.D., in her book *Nutrition for Vegetarians,* "Any drug that will stimulate the nerves will stimulate the appetite in susceptible people. This includes coffee, tea, colas, and chocolate. These beverages stimulate cravings."

If you consume beverages that contain caffeine, pay attention to the ways they affect your attitude and your appetite. You may decide to discontinue or moderate your use and try herbal teas, sparkling mineral water, and natural spritzers (mineral water and fruit juice) instead. The drink that helped get a diet-cola hankering the size of Texas off my back is licorice tea. Hot or iced, this herbal drink is naturally sweet but calorically negligible.

With animal products, junk foods, and iffy drinks out of your diet, you'll also have inadvertently eliminated all or most of your personal binge foods. You may, however, have others, and it's important that you come to terms with them. Not everyone who wants to lose a few pounds has binge foods, but if you've ever been on an eating binge—that's an all-out food frenzy that leaves you feeling intoxicated—you're probably intimately acquainted with them. People describe binge-inciting foods as "better than sex" and say that "one bite is too many and a thousand aren't enough." These are the foods that encourage appetite instead of extinguishing it. You really can't eat just one. If you have some today, you'll need more tomorrow. In other words, binge foods are addictive.

The usual recipe for a binge food is fat plus sugar or fat plus salt. Common culprits, then, are what you'd expect: ice cream, chips, chocolate, pastries, and cheese. But even something as subtle as combining nuts and raisins for trail mix can turn two otherwise innocuous foods into the makings of some overeater's lost weekend. Besides, binge foods are intensely personal. For a given individual, something about the taste or texture of almost any food, or past associations with it, can make it far more than just something to eat. You may have trouble with a broad category of foods—sugar, meat, flour, or anything at your mom's house—or specific items such as granola, yogurt, dates, peanut butter, or white bread.

If you can be really honest with yourself, you'll probably realize that you already know your own red-light foods. You may not want to claim them, but you may as well—they've already claimed you. If you're unsure about a specific suspect, try to eat a little and save the rest for next week. If you can't do it, or if you think incessantly about it while it sits in the cupboard or fridge, you have yourself a binge food.

The point in identifying these is to protect yourself from infiltrators out to sabotage your victory. If there was a stalker set on harming you, you'd notify the police and do everything in your power to protect yourself. Understand that any food you haven't been able to eat reasonably since you cut teeth is as threatening to you as that stalker. The safest path to tread with a binge food is the one that leads away from it. In other words, don't eat it—not because I said so, but because you'd rather not socialize with a dietary hit man.

The prospect of living without some food you've depended on may seem unbearable, but you can do it. The secret is to think in terms of *today* instead of eternity. There's disagreement among eating-disorders experts and recovering overeaters (who are also experts, in my opinion) on whether or not these dynamite foods can ever be defused. That is to say, can the allure of carrot cake come down to that of carrot sticks? I've found that I'm able to eat anything that I choose to eat today providing my spiritual life is in order. Other overeaters in recovery—people every bit as attentive to their spiritual lives as I am—assiduously avoid certain foods, usually sweets.

With the Twelve-Steppers' trio of honesty, open-mindedness, and willingness, you'll find your own way with binge foods. They are potentially loaded weapons, but they will in time lose much of their attractiveness. One of these days, you'll find yourself looking at a onetime temptation as if it were an old flame and thinking, "What did I ever see in that one?"

Snacking—with wild abandon at least—can meet a similar fate. With the love-powered diet, you can elect to snack on something that will support your health, or you may decide not to snack at all. There are magazine articles all the time claiming that eating small, frequent meals (snacking or "grazing") keeps blood sugar steady and is therefore superior to having three regular meals. This works for certain people and there are, in fact, medical conditions that require it. For most of us, though, the sanest approach is also the simplest: three reasonable meals a day, eaten on a fairly predictable schedule. As I first put it in my book *Fit from Within*: "If you

Nourished by Love

. . . .

- *Choose natural foods from the plant kingdom—fruits, vegetables, whole grains, and legumes.* If you aren't ready to become a complete vegetarian, use animal foods more for variety and flavor than as major players.

- *Know that plant foods may be eaten generously.* Have ample portions from the four plant-based food groups (fruits, vegetables, whole grains, and legumes) and use concentrated sweets and oil-rich foods sparingly. If you enjoy salad, eat all you want; just keep an eye on the amount of dressing you're using.

- *Avoid second helpings as a general rule.* When you serve yourself, start with enough. If someone serves you a piddling portion, have more.

- *Rethink the main course.* Make sure that rice, potatoes, or a large salad with pasta or beans in it can fit there. Round out meals with more vegetables, whole-grain bread, and so forth.

- *Use rich foods like nuts, avocado, and dried fruit sparingly.* (If you're healthy and don't need to lose weight or can handle the extra calories, you can eat more of these.)

- *Go for quality.* You deserve better than junk food. For the most part, leave sugar, grease, and excess salt on their side of the tracks—the wrong side. Caffeine and alcohol consumption should be reduced or eliminated.

- *As a rule, have three meals a day unless you have a health condition that requires you to eat more often.* Sit down during meals. Have a place setting. Try not to rush through the meal. Keep it nice: argue some other time. And don't watch TV at mealtime.

- *If you want a snack, have fruit, raw veggies, or freshly extracted juice such as carrot/celery/spinach or kale/romaine/apple/lemon.* Feeling hungry—not faint, not shaky, just hungry—for a while before a meal is OK, too.

- *Eat only when you're emotionally and spiritually centered.* If you feel that you're about to eat for a fix, even at mealtime, get yourself together first by calling a supportive friend, taking a walk, or writing in your journal.

- *Avoid personal binge foods.* These are the foods that seem to incite overeating or that you obsess over when they're around. A love-powered diet eliminates most of the common ones, but recognize and respect yours, common or not.

- *Leave a little food on your plate.* I've heard it called the *angel bite*. You're

Nourished by Love (*continued*)

. . . .

not a failure when you don't do this, but you get lots of inner nourishment when you do.

- *Follow the "Nutritional Guidelines" below.* Familiarize yourself with the fundamental nutritional information in Chapter Seven, "Healthy and Whole," and help ensure your general health with the suggestions in Chapter Nine, "Love-Powered Living."

- *Give less power to the scale.* Find a sensible midpoint between frequent weighing and refusing to find out what you weigh. Decide to weigh yourself once or twice a month and stay with that. You will lose weight. Give yourself an edge with exercise. If you have a history of crash dieting, or if you have been bulimic, it may take time for your body to respond to normal, healthful eating with the loss of weight you're looking for. Be patient. Concentrate on self-acceptance and on enjoying the day at hand.

  Remember that you're working with the laws of nature. They can't be rushed and they can't be cheated. Allow yourself to be a part of the natural process. This is for life, so there's no reason to hurry. Don't be discouraged by a slow-moving scale. If you want to be impressed by a number, look at your love-powered cholesterol level.

- *Get the help you need.* Continue to ask God (or whatever you call your Higher Power) each morning for help in eating reasonably that day. Say thanks at night, even if your eating wasn't perfect. Attend Overeaters Anonymous meetings in person, online, and on the phone. Read the books and visit the websites listed at the back of this book.

- *Give yourself priority status.* Allow yourself time for meals and food preparation, for meditation, exercise, support group meetings, and whatever else you need. This isn't selfishness— it's self-preservation.

start to eat only three times, you have to stop only three times, and stopping has been the problem."

In the earliest stages of your lifestyle change, you may need large meals to bridge the gap between binge eating and moderation. That's fine. Begin wherever you can. With a commitment to three meals, you'll find that you'll have the opportunity to experience hours without eating. You'll learn to conduct your life without a snack at hand. Moreover, society is set up for three meals a day. You go on vacation and stay at a bed-and-breakfast. Your workday is punctuated with a lunch hour. You're invited out for dinner.

As you embark on this adventure, you'll be enjoying bountiful meals and may well find that eating three of these a day with nothing but living in between is fully adequate. On the other hand, this is a low-fat food plan that includes lots of water-rich fruits and vegetables that are efficiently processed by your digestive apparatus. They don't stay with you like heavy, fatty foods that must be laboriously digested. Therefore, you may feel the need for something to eat at morning break time, or in the middle of the afternoon, or before bed.

The best snack is a piece of fruit. This is the original, portable fast food. The natural sugars in fruit will pick up your energy, and it's as close to fat-free as you're going to get. Have fruit between meals if you want it. Raw vegetables make good snacks, too, and it's good to keep them washed, chopped, and ready. Freshly extracted vegetable juices, especially those that include the nutrient superstars, dark, leafy greens, may well be the best snack going. They flood your system with needed nutrition and lasting satisfaction in liquid form, so the noshing reflex—a nibble here, a nibble there—isn't activated. (They make a terrific beverage with meals as well.)

In any event, you never have to go hungry. You may at times choose to feel hungry, and that's all right, too. Oh, I know that no book like this is supposed to suggest that you'll ever feel any less satiated than a just-nursed infant, but that isn't realistic. Mom doesn't pack us lunches anymore, and there will be times when we would like to eat and will need to wait. Saying no sometimes is as much a part of the privilege of adulthood as saying yes.

This is where flexibility comes in—flexibility in your food plan and your thinking. When you're spiritually fit, you can make rational decisions, even when those decisions are about food. Let's say that you have to dash to the airport to catch a flight without having supper. All you see at the kiosk near your flight gate are candy bars and salted peanuts. You have choices. You can buy a candy bar—ideally a healthy, vegan one like a Lara bar or a Luna bar—or some peanuts. Or you can choose to feel a little hungry and wait until more substantial food is available. What would you do? I'd get the Lara bar. Even though I generally stick with fresh fruit, juice, or nothing at all between meals, this is a perfectly legitimate action in a less-than-perfect situation.

You have to make this a way of life that works for you in the real world, *your* real world. I can tell you that it's worked for me for over twenty years as I've traveled for business and pleasure all over the country and around the world. I had no problems in Tibet or Iceland, and only a few on the Interstate in my native Missouri.

Generous, Delicious, and Aesthetically Pleasing

One downside of dieting is a lack of food. You're told to compensate by using a smaller plate. Now you can use a standard plate and a big salad bowl. If a substantial salad with a light dressing is the center of your meal, ordinary salad bowls are a joke. Uncooked vegetables as well as fruits are both low in fat and high in water; therefore they are low in calories. The filling starches from which you'll make many of your entrées—rice, pasta, beans, potatoes (yes, plural!)—are low-fat foods as well, so they're lower in calories than traditional main dishes.

Even the leaner animal foods are generally higher in fat than grains, vegetables, and most beans. In addition, some evidence suggests that calories from fat are more fattening than the same number of calories from carbohydrates, because the body has to work to turn carbs into storable fat while dietary fat can be stored as is.

I'm not suggesting that because most love-powered foods won't put you at odds with the bathroom scale, you should overeat. I *am* saying, however, that the concept of a moderate portion has to be redefined when you adopt a low-fat diet. If you're having salad, steamed asparagus, and corn on the cob for dinner, don't have one ear of corn: have a couple, and a whole-wheat roll, too, if you want it (just spread on some all-fruit jam and bypass the margarine or butter). You'll need to re-think portion sizes on the side dishes that, in this way of eating, become entrées. Those boxes of rice pilaf, for example, don't serve six anymore. They served six with roast beef. As a main course, they'll serve two or three.

Not only are love-powered portions generous, the variety of foods from which you'll choose is enormous. When people find out that you're doing this, they'll say,

"But what do you eat?" Take it from me: they wouldn't stand still long enough to hear the names of all the tasty foods on nature's table. (See Chapter Eight, "Food for Life" for lists of some of the many foods you'll enjoy.)

When you're eating natural foods and concentrating on those from the plant kingdom, you'll become more aware of seasonal fruits and vegetables. When you travel, you'll find regional delights that are lost to people on the burger-and-fries circuit. There are hundreds of varieties of vegetables and fruits, dozens of kinds of grains and legumes, and plenty of interesting specialty and convenience foods made from them.

From this abundance, you can select what you like. You don't have to eat any specific food—not grapefruit, not spinach, not soybeans. You build your eating plan around foods you already like, and with a little daring you can discover both delicious new foods and tasty new ways to fix old favorites.

Either way, what you'll offer yourself and others to eat will look beautiful. A supermarket checker once bagged my week's provisions and said, "I've had this job for fifteen years and I've never seen such pretty groceries!" That's because fruits and vegetables really are edible works of art, and whether in a shopping cart or on a serving tray, they are very appealing to people. Natural foods from the plant kingdom entice the eye and have wonderful fragrances and distinctive flavors. They tantalize several senses, and meals based on them invite appreciation and the slower pace that's essential in retraining eating habits.

It's also pleasant to be in the company of these foods. If you were going to meet a friend in the city, wouldn't you rather rendezvous at a fruit stand than at a butcher shop or fish market? And if you went back to your place for the kind of simple but elegant dinner you'll soon be adept at preparing, cleanup would be a breeze. Greasy pots do not exist when you don't fix greasy foods, and that counts as aesthetically pleasing, too.

Eating for High-Level Health *and* Normal Weight

"I have lived quite long enough and am trying to die," wrote vegetarian George Bernard Shaw at 84, "but I simply cannot do it. A single beefsteak would finish

93

Nutritional Guidelines

. . . .

A love-powered food plan provides optimum nutrition for your health. Following these guidelines will further ensure that. If you're under a doctor's care, consult him or her about your eating plan.

If you're pregnant or nursing, follow the advice of your health care provider. Also visit www.pcrm.org/health/veginfo/-pregnancy.html for nutritional information for a vegan pregnancy from Physicians Committee for Responsible Medicine; read the excellent article "Pregnancy and the Vegan Diet," by Reed Mangels, Ph.D., RD, available on the Vegetarian Resource Group's website (www.vrg.org); or visit vegfamily.com/vegan-pregnancy.

1. Eat from the four main love-powered food groups daily: vegetables, fruits, whole grains, and legumes. Use of some healthy fats—nuts and seeds, avocado, a little olive and flax oil—is also fine; just don't overdo. If you wish to continue using some animal products for now, keep your intake moderate and have a plan for making the break for good.

2. Enjoy at least one large salad every day and include in it a variety of leafy greens (romaine, leaf lettuce, spinach) plus other vegetables. Include foods rich in vitamin C such as citrus fruits, cantaloupe, bell peppers, tomatoes, and strawberries.

3. Eat foods with a high vitamin C content along with iron-rich foods. This helps increase iron absorption by your body. High-iron foods include beans, peas, and lentils; dried fruit such as prunes and figs; almonds and cashews; whole grains; and leafy greens (the greens come with their own vitamin C).

4. Include at least two daily servings of calcium-rich foods such as collards, kale, broccoli, oatmeal, soybeans, tofu cultured with calcium sulfate, almonds, sesame seeds or tahini (sesame-seed butter), calcium-fortified orange juice, or calcium-fortified soymilk or rice milk. Virtually all your food will provide some calcium, and much research indicates that people need less of this mineral on a plant-based diet than on one high in animal protein.

5. Be sure to get vitamin D through moderate exposure to sunlight. While this is of particular concern to dark-skinned people living in northern latitudes, recent research suggests that vitamin D deficiency is widespread. Most nutritionists now recommend taking supplementary vitamin D, up to 400 IU daily.

Nutritional Guidelines (*continued*)

. . . .

6. Supplement your diet regularly with a source of vitamin B12 (cobalamin) to meet the Daily Value of six micrograms. B12 tablets contain more than this and may be taken weekly. Many vegetarian foods are fortified with B12, including some meat analogs, nutritional yeasts, fortified soymilk, and some commonly available cereals (check the label). (For more on B12 see Chapter Seven, "Healthy and Whole.")

7. For a plethora of disease-preventing phytochemicals think *color* and eat a rainbow of foods: blueberries, tomatoes, pumpkin and squash, kale and collards, watermelon. Also include a vegetable from the cabbage family (broccoli, Brussels sprouts, cauliflower) on your menu at least four times a week.

8. Don't overdo protein by eating too many beans—a cup a day is plenty. The love-powered diet will keep your protein intake at the proper level. Provided you obtain adequate calories from a variety of natural foods, you'll secure ample protein without special foods or food combinations.

9. Be moderate in your use of nuts, seeds, olives, and avocado, and be ever so sparing in your use of oil for cooking and in salad dressings to keep fat consumption low. Cut down by water-sautéing, substituting applesauce for shortening in baking, and using non-stick cookware. (For more information on low-fat recipe substitutions, see "Fat Zappers" in Chapter Eight.) Even so, if you eat a plant-based diet, it will automatically be fairly low in total fat and very low in artery-clogging saturated fat.

me, but I cannot bring myself to swallow it. I am oppressed with a dread of living forever. That is the only disadvantage of vegetarianism."

While no diet can substitute for longevity genes, a poor diet can keep you from reaching your potential for both quality and length of life. Here are statistics reported by John Robbins in his classic, *Diet for a New America*:

- The average American man has a fifty percent chance of dying from a heart attack; the average total vegetarian man reduces that risk to four percent.

- No country in the world with a high intake of meat has a low incidence of colon cancer.
- Women who eat eggs three or more days a week, compared to less than once a week, have a three times greater risk of developing fatal ovarian cancer.
- Men who consume meats, dairy products, and eggs daily, as compared to sparingly, run a 3.6 times greater risk of developing fatal prostate cancer.
- The average measurable bone loss of female meat-eaters at age sixty-five is thirty-five percent; in vegetarian women it is eighteen percent.

A variety of factors may account for the apparent superiority of a vegetarian or near-vegetarian diet. In replacing animal foods with unrefined grains, fruits, vegetables, and legumes, a dietary program results that is:

- Cholesterol-free (cholesterol in our diets comes only from foods of animal origin)
- Low in fats, especially saturated fats
- High in natural carbohydrates (don't panic: these are whole, natural carbs that will keep you going, not fatten you up)
- Rich in fiber
- Abundant in vitamins A and C, which some research indicates may protect against certain cancers, and other possible anti-carcinogens such as indoles in cruciferous (cabbage family) vegetables and protease inhibitors in legumes
- Adequate but not excessive in protein (too much protein has been linked with osteoporosis, kidney stones, and deterioration of kidney function)
- Markedly lower in pesticide residues, particularly chlorinated hydrocarbons, than are animal foods (these residues concentrate in the fatty tissues of animals)
- Bulky and satisfying to assuage hunger without excess calories

It's widely accepted, therefore, in medical literature that vegans—people who eat only plant foods and no meat, fish, eggs, or dairy products—typically weigh eight to twenty pounds less than comparable omnivores, who average seventeen to twenty-two pounds over ideal weight. The serendipitous thing about vegans and weight is that their slimness is not something they work at. It happens naturally—without hunger, suffering, or willpower. That's precisely how it will happen for you, provided that you practice the spiritual principles that will keep you from needing to eat for a fix, and that you build your diet predominantly from the love-powered food groups.

Economical Eating with Plenty for All

You can afford a love-powered diet, even if you're a full-time student, a retired person on a fixed income, or a food-stamp recipient. The staples for this eating style are among the most inexpensive foods in the marketplace: brown rice, beans, whole-wheat flour and bread, potatoes, carrots, greens and other seasonal vegetables, apples, oranges, bananas, and other fruits selected when they're most abundant and least costly. And you can grow nutritious sprouts on a kitchen counter—alfalfa, mung beans, sunflower . . . the list is endless—for mere pennies. (See the "Sprout Farming" section in Chapter Eight.) You'll be saving cash by skipping the high-ticket items like meat and cheese—as well as the junk foods, which may sometimes be bargains until you consider the physiological price you pay for them.

You certainly can spend money on rare, tropical fruits, exotic vegetables (I'm astounded by how many vegetables come in purple), health food store convenience items, and gourmet specialties. You don't need these, though, to design love-powered menus that are nutritious and conducive to bringing your best body into being. Simple foods—those that the planet provides generously for all—can be the makings of elegant repasts, celebrations of life and health in good taste and good conscience.

A Way of Eating that Respects All Life

In summer and fall, the classifieds are filled with ads for "pick-your-own" places, inviting city folks on country outings that will bring in a miniature harvest of apples or berries. That's the same time of year that the gardeners are out in force, turning suburban yards into small truck farms or greening midtown balconies with lettuce and radish and tomato plants. People delight in these pursuits, even before the fruits of their labors reach the dinner table.

Throughout the year, however, something else is going on. Animals are being slaughtered for us to eat. We usually don't stop to think that a Kansas City steak was recently a Kansas cow, but as philosopher Peter Singer wrote in his seminal work *Animal Liberation*, "For most humans, especially those in modern urban and suburban communities, the most direct form of contact with nonhuman animals is at mealtime. We eat them."

And the number of animals we eat is, according to Physicians Committee for Responsible Medicine, an astronomical nine-billion-plus every year. That comes to *one million per hour*. If you think of each of these beings as *an individual*, like the pig or sheep you would take your child to meet at an animal sanctuary or petting zoo, knowledge of this daily holocaust can come like a kick in the stomach.

Many people believe that this is simply the way life is supposed to work—survival of the fittest, dominion over everybody, top-of-the-food-chain, etc. People used similar arguments to justify slavery, child labor, and genocide, and in too many parts of the world, they still do. In those cases, as in this one, these aren't arguments, they're smokescreens. While you need not be a vegetarian to develop the spiritual connection that will free you from the need to abuse food, maintaining that connection does ask that you take responsibility for your actions. Would you, in an ordinary, non-emergency situation, kill an animal and eat it? Most people find the prospect repugnant—quite unlike picking apples or growing tomato plants.

In fact, most people I know support the killing of animals for meat through their food choices, yet when I asked *fifteen of them* if they would go with me when I had the rare opportunity to tour a slaughterhouse, they refused one at a time. I went by myself.

While the entire experience lives in my brain as a real-life horror movie complete with the cold, the blood, the screams, the stench, and deplorable conditions for the workers, there was one cow whose face, and fate, will be etched in my memory until I take my last breath. She was old, a reject from a dairy herd—"used up," the man said. She seemed comfortable with people and trusting, so she didn't require the cattle prod—an instrument capable of producing first-degree burns—to walk the

In Case You May Be Wondering . . .

. . . .

Where will I get my protein? We'll cover this in detail in the upcoming chapter, and there's even more info in Appendix B, "Nutshell Nutrition." Know for now that, despite all you've heard, it's easy to get adequate protein on a natural, plant-based diet, provided you eat a variety of foods and obtain adequate calories.

I used to be a vegetarian but it didn't agree with me. What kind of vegetarian were you? Did you eat junk food? Did you eat a lot of cheese and other dairy products? If so, your diet was not what I'm recommending in this book.

Also, did you consider your personal needs and make adaptations accordingly? For example, even though whole grains play an important role in the diet of most vegetarians and vegans, some people have a hard time digesting them. There are vegetarians who have to be careful about what grains they eat: many stay away from gluten-containing grains (wheat, rye, oats, and spelt) but do well with lighter grains such as millet, quinoa, and amaranth. Some vegetarians, including most raw-fooders, don't eat grains at all and do fine.

There are individuals who have a problem with another vegetarian staple, soy. For all the good it does the rest of us, it just doesn't sit well with certain people.

If you're one of them, you can absolutely be a soy-free vegan. This will limit your choice of prepared foods but it will not keep you from having a nutritious and delicious diet.

If you want to go veg again, think of all the important reasons why you're doing it, and why it deserves to be a lifetime commitment. Help it be that by honoring yourself and listening to your body. You may also want to enlist the help of a vegan physician or dietitian in formulating a way of eating that makes you feel like a million bucks. Some websites to start with are www.drfuhrman.com and www.drmcdougall.com.

Can't I just do this part way? You can do it part way, all the way, three-quarters of the way, or not at all. You have complete autonomy. I am presenting you with what I've found to be a beautiful way to live and flourish, free from obsession. I believe it to be a plan that will help you lose weight, be satisfied, enjoy your food, keep the weight off, and have a life of so much depth and meaning that eating for a fix will one day be only a memory. If transitioning to a plant-based diet seems like too much for you to do all at once, do it gradually.

Maybe you'll want to drop the cruelest foods first—veal, *foie gras*, and factory-

In Case You May Be Wondering . . . (*continued*)

. . . .

farmed eggs. After a few weeks, you can work up to all meat and poultry. This leaves you with fish and dairy. Save the fish for when you eat out. This means that at home you're a lacto-vegetarian. Give that some time. Get used to it. See how you do. Be careful that you don't overdo cheese during this phase since it's a binge food for a lot of people and it's easy for almost anyone to overeat cheese. Otherwise, you can go pretty easy on yourself.

Do this for a while—say, six months. Keep educating yourself along the way. Invest in some vegan cookbooks (there are many recommendations in Appendix C) and discover what great stuff you're able to make. Note the changes in the way you do things and the way you feel. After six months, regroup and reconsider. How hard would it be now to swap your skim milk for rice milk, almond milk, or low-fat soy? How about choosing a vegan entrée instead of all that fish when you go out? Chances are, you'll already be making these choices much of the time and taking the step to vegan won't seem like such a big one. You may look back and say, "You know what? I could have done this overnight."

I'm not supposed to eat like this because I have the blood type that needs meat.

The blood type theory (A's can be vegetarian, B's are in between, O's must eat meat) is not based on solid science and has been thoroughly debunked. Vegetarians of every blood type are alive and well.

The only meat I eat now is the humanely raised kind. Good for you for taking that step. I invite you to go farther. You see, so-called humanely raised farm animals should, at least in theory, have a better life that those confined to the living-hell conditions of an all-out factory farm. However, these initiatives aren't legally binding. The farmer (usually not the family farmer in your kids' storybooks, but a giant conglomerate) makes the rules. Concessions for the animals' comfort are often minor and of course the horror of the slaughterhouse ends the story.

Also, what I see in practice is that people who conscientiously choose the humane labels when they shop eat whatever is on the menu when they go out or dine at other people's homes, thereby diluting whatever benefit may have come from their original choice. And there are still the problems of environmental devastation and your own health to contend with. Taking the leap and going vegetarian—ideally all the way to a love-powered vegan diet—makes more sense (and it really isn't that hard).

In Case You May Be Wondering . . . (*continued*)

. . . .

Would it count if I ate meat but said thank you to the animal that sacrificed its life, like the Native Americans? Whenever I hear this, I imagine, heaven forbid, someone holding a gun to my head and telling me that he appreciated my sacrifice and that he'll pray for me after I'm dead. I don't think that would cancel out the fact that he was about to do me in.

Seriously, I respect Native American tradition and in a subsistence culture where hunting was necessary for survival, the idea of honoring the murdered animal was admirable. But you don't live in a culture like that. You have supermarkets and Whole Foods and Jamba Juice. In other words, you eat meat because you want to. I think you'd be better off if you didn't. I know the animals would be. But it's your choice. Read the information presented here and go with the guidance of your own mind and heart.

I really like the spiritual, Twelve Step stuff. What if I just do that and find my own way to eat? You're certainly free to do that. In fact, if you were to go to a meeting of Overeaters Anonymous, you'd find most of the people doing that very thing. What I'm offering you in this book is a way to bring your spiritual principles full circle and have them operative in every area of your life, particularly as they apply to food. When you add humane dietary principles to your spiritual practice, you'll find that your practice deepens (why do you think most yogis and Trappist monks are vegetarian?) and your life daily becomes more meaningful and more complete.

---

ramp to the metal enclosure where she would be stunned with the captive bolt pistol. When the worker came at her with the stunner, she crouched to avoid it. He whistled at her, the way I imagined he might whistle at his dog when he got home that evening. She raised her head in response and was shot with the captive bolt.

She dropped to the floor, was immediately hoisted up by one leg, her throat slit, and as the blood gushed from her body, she was efficiently skinned before my eyes. She was turned within a minute, maybe two, from *being* to *beef*. "You have just dined," wrote Ralph Waldo Emerson, "and however scrupulously the slaughterhouse is concealed in the distance of miles, there is complicity." Emerson was a vegetarian.

Today there are problems in the barnyard as well as at the slaughterhouse. Most of the animals raised for food today come from factory farms where they may be confined to small cages or stalls, and without anesthesia are dehorned, de-tailed, de-beaked, and mutilated in other ways. Many are denied exercise, companionship, natural diets, and other basic needs, and there are no federal laws protecting them. Even animals whose rearing supposedly meets certain "compassion standards" are commodities. Male chicks are killed soon after birth, even in so-called free-range egg operations. Mother cows in dairy herds are separated from their babies—and male calves usually killed for veal—on even "organic" dairy farms.

It could be argued that some animal foods come with a higher pain cost than others, and many people who aren't vegetarian but whose compassion has been aroused by information have stopped eating certain foods. Among these are:

- *Foie gras*, the "fatty liver" from ducks and geese that some gourmets foolishly prize, is the result of sadistic force-feeding that results in a diseased liver and an expensive appetizer. *Foie gras* is banned in several countries and was even decried by Pope Benedict.
- Veal is another item on the cruelty menu. Calves are taken from their dairy-cow mothers shortly after birth—a horrible separation for both. They are confined in crates in which they cannot turn around, and fed an anemic diet to preserve the babyish white flesh. Although there's some movement toward "less intensive" veal operations, there's none yet that would invite a fifth grade class for a field trip.
- Factory-farmed eggs are another ugly story—one that, like the slaughterhouse, I can tell firsthand because I've been to the "batteries" where they're produced. Male chicks are of no use in an egg operation so they're killed, often by suffocation or shredding, soon after hatching. The females, de-beaked and de-clawed, are crammed into tiny cages allowing them no social interaction or any semblance of a normal life. Many die daily and one worker at a "farm" I visited had as his job to remove the dead birds every morning.

Although these are among the more horrific stories, agribusiness is *one indus-*

try and using animals for food opens the way for abuses. If, for example, there were no demand for dairy, there would be no veal industry. While consideration for the animals involved may never be your motivation for a diet that excludes animal foods, expect that as you adopt some of the principles found here your overall reverence for life will expand. You may not interpret or express that reverence in the way that someone else might, but expect to see it in your life because it will be there. As psychologist Virginia Satir wrote, "Spiritual power can be seen in a person's reverence for life—hers and all others, including animals and nature, with a recognition of a universal life force referred to by many as God."

Food for a Sustainable Planet

This way of eating is as gentle to the Earth as it is to animals and arteries. Eating low on the food chain (i.e., a plant-based diet) can be just as easy to incorporate into an ecologically aware lifestyle as other responsible practices like recycling cans and recharging batteries.

Why a diet that doesn't depend on animal foods is vital in restoring health to an ailing planet is explained in the following facts and figures from John Robbins:

- About seventy-five percent of U.S. topsoil has been lost to date, and eighty-five percent of U.S. topsoil loss is directly associated with the raising of livestock.
- Some 260 million acres of U.S. forests have been cleared for cropland to produce a meat-centered diet.
- Every individual who switches to a complete vegetarian diet saves an acre of trees each year.
- About thirty-three percent of all raw materials (base products of farming, forestry, and mining, including fossil fuels) consumed by the United States are devoted to the production of livestock.
- More than half the water used for all purposes in the United States goes for livestock production.
- Livestock in this country produce 230,000 pounds of excrement every second. Feedlots don't have sewage systems, so with every rainstorm a part of the one bil-

lion tons of waste generated annually in confinement operations goes into streams, rivers, and groundwater.

- To get a single calorie of protein from beef requires seventy-eight calories of fossil fuel. One calorie of protein from soybeans requires just two calories of fossil fuel.

A 2006 report from the United Nations Food and Agriculture Organization states that animal agriculture is responsible for eighteen percent of greenhouse gas emissions. *That's more than is attributable to all our cars, trucks, and SUVs.*

Statistics can be numbing and the whole notion of an environmental crisis can seem so overwhelming that the very thought of it can push a shut-off valve in our psyches to divert our thinking elsewhere. True, the Earth's ills are enormous and it will take action on myriad fronts to heal them. Contributing to the wellbeing of the planet with Earth-loving food choices is one such action, one which takes no time and no extraordinary effort. You're probably busy with all sorts of things, but you'll stop for lunch, and making it a love-powered meal can be an effortless donation to a most deserving planet.

In addition to the environmental benefits brought about by eating low on the food chain, there are subtler ways in which simpler eating supports an ecological ethic. Since you'll be selecting natural foods, many of which can be bought in bulk and put in reusable containers, you'll be using fewer packaging materials. You'll be less likely to visit fast-food places with their plethora of disposables, and since you won't have meat scraps, all of your garbage can be composted. With the money you save, you can buy some food that's organically grown, and with more fresh fruits and salads in your diet, you may use your stove less often and save energy. Also, this is clean eating; you'll have fewer dishes to wash so you'll use less detergent and hot water.

A love-powered diet may also cause the environmentalist within you to emerge by inviting nature into your kitchen. Don't be surprised if you find yourself growing parsley and chives in clay pots on your windowsills or raising a crop of alfalfa sprouts on your counter. You might even find yourself planting a tree that, in a few years or several, will bear fruit or nuts. When this was suggested to me, I argued,

"Why should I plant a fruit tree? I won't even be living in this house when it gets its first peach." But "Someone will be living there," I was reminded. A tree, then, can be a contribution to strangers and the Earth. And eating from trees, gardens, and fields can be a gift to yourself, one of all sorts of ways that you'll discover to make the love in your life practical and viable.

CHAPTER SEVEN

HEALTHY AND WHOLE

In order to confidently make the change to a plant-based diet—to plan meals that will best support your health, and answer the questions you're sure to be asked when people see that you're eating differently—you'll need some information. The purpose of this chapter is to help you learn more about vegetarian nutrition. In addition, there's a basic primer on general nutrition, "Nutrition in a Nutshell," in the back of this book.

People are very trusting when it comes to nourishing their bodies. Oh, we can sound pretty sophisticated talking about amino acids and omega-3s, but don't you think most people believe that anything on a grocer's shelf that doesn't have a skull and crossbones on it is at least suitable for human consumption? Most folks pride themselves on being omnivores: "I can eat anything" and "I have a cast-iron stomach," we boast. Nevertheless, the results of eating everything edible and treating our stomachs as if they were indeed formed in a smelter are devastating.

We see these results in obesity, digestive disorders, and degenerative disease. What's more, this seems normal. Repeated diets, popping antacids, even submitting to major surgery are practices so common they're regarded as inevitable. This simpler way of eating, although not a panacea, may be an alternative. When introduced to it, however, people often respond defensively. They want to know, "Where do you get your protein? Where do you get your calcium? Where do you get your iron?" The answer is that all these nutrients come to us from the plant kingdom. By eating plant foods, we get them directly. With animal foods, we get them secondhand.

Still, most people eat everything and assume that doing so is essential for good health. That assumption has been substantiated over the years with the assorted caveats applied to vegetarian diets. These include such assertions as: "It's all right not to eat meat, but you need to have plenty of milk and eggs and maybe some fish every so often"; and "Vegetarians need to take lots of supplements"; and "You can only eat that way if you combine your food just right and plan every meal very carefully."

I'll bet even skydivers and hang-glider pilots don't get such persistent warnings. To top it off, not one of these arguments has an actual basis in current scientific information. On the contrary, natural vegetarian foods are generally rich in nutritional value, largely low in fat, and absolutely free of cholesterol, so a lot of the "balancing" that we think of as necessary in designing any food plan is taken care of with this simple choice.

This is one important reason why a plant-based diet can be a helpful tool for keeping food obsession from resurfacing: you don't have to spend an inordinate amount of time thinking about your food. Natural vegetarian meals are complete and nourishing. Your body knows what to do with them so you can stop counting, quantifying, measuring, and worrying about what you eat. You can put your mind on other things.

What's So SAD about the Standard American Diet?

The prestigious journals of medicine and nutrition have for decades been dotted with reports connecting the way people eat with many of the ills they endure. A great many of these studies show that vegetarian or near-vegetarian diets can reduce the risk for many of the diseases and disorders that plague modern society. Apparently, several key differences exist between a natural vegetarian diet and the standard American diet. A way of eating based on plant foods is naturally low in fat, high in fiber, and moderate in protein. The typical American diet, on the other hand, is built around animal foods and is high in fat, deficient in fiber, and excessive in protein.

The SAD Is Built around Animal Foods

Michael Klaper, M.D., makes the straightforward declaration: "The body of *Homo sapiens* has no nutritional requirement for the flesh of animals, for the eggs of chickens or for the milk of cows." Not only can we be well-nourished without them, there's ample evidence that such foods are actually harmful. In addition to the load of cholesterol, fat, and protein in most of them and their dearth of fiber, animal foods are also the major dietary source of purines, which cause a rise in fat and glucose levels in the blood—a rise likely to encourage fat storage in the body. Meats are deficient in carbohydrate, the food component that should account for sixty to eighty percent of the calories ingested. (Carbohydrate-deficient diets lead to decreased endurance. If you want to up your exercise, you need to be eating good carbs.)

Because the levels of toxins in animal foods are much higher than those in plants (in some studies, sixteen times higher), eating plants instead of animals greatly reduces intake of these poisons. Of course, choosing organic produce can also result in a marked decrease in the amount of synthetic pesticides consumed. Even so, it's believed that the average person ingests far more of these in animal products than in vegetable foods.

And pesticide residues aren't the only extras in a slab of steak or bucket of chicken. Growth hormones are commonly used in livestock production, and fifty-five percent of the antibiotics used in the United States are routinely fed to animals on farms. This is believed to have contributed to the noticeable rise in antibiotic-resistant infections over the past forty years. Stress hormones secreted by the animal prior to slaughter also become a part of the meat.

Wild fish, too, although not intentionally fed potential toxins by humans, are subject to the effects of chemical runoff in our rivers, lakes, and seas. Although many people who are otherwise vegetarian choose to include some fish in their diets and seem to do so successfully, it's nevertheless a fact that many fish show serious concentrations of heavy metals, mutation-inducing hydrocarbons, and radioactivity from nuclear pollution.

The SAD Is High in Fat

The typical Western diet—rapidly being exported around the world—relies on meats, fish, eggs, and dairy products, along with fried foods and rich baked goods. It provides too much fat—thirty-six percent of calories on average—as well as artery-clogging cholesterol. Fats carry calories at more than double the amount of either proteins or carbohydrates (nine calories per gram for fat, four for proteins and carbs). In other words, eating fat means getting more calories from less food. Eating enough high-fat foods to feel full is likely to lead to weight gain, but cutting portion sizes to include these foods results in leaving the table hungry—the first step in the demise of one more diet.

Because the media likes new and revolutionary ideas, it had a great run with low-fat foods in the 1980s and early 1990s when the health problems with diets high in fat began to surface. Once low-fat was no longer hot, the trend swung back to recommendations for more protein in the diet and a loosening up on concern about fat. Trends aside, human physiology didn't change. It's as difficult right now for the body to deal with an onslaught of fat—and, for that matter, with too much protein—as it ever was.

It's true that when low-fat and fat-free foods became a cash cow for food manufacturers, lots of people went in for orgies of overeating on concentrated sweets and other manufactured products simply because the packages proclaimed their fat-free status. Some people ate so many fat-free cookies and crackers and cakes that they actually gained weight. This kind of foolishness doesn't negate the basic reality that excess fat is harmful to health and that a low-fat diet based on real food—not mass-produced junk food, whether high or low in fat—is ideal.

Not only do fats have more calories than other foods, the body likes to hang on to calories from fat. It's a physiological principle that many of the excess calories from carbohydrates are stored in the liver as glycogen so they can be drawn upon for use as energy. The evidence strongly suggests, however, that fats ingested in foods can be appropriated for body fat much more easily.

Animal foods have, as a rule, a much higher fat content than do vegetables, fruits, grains, and legumes. In addition, animal fats are of a different type than vegetable fats. They are primarily saturated, and it's saturated fat that plays a part in elevating blood cholesterol levels. (A few plant foods—primarily tropical oils such as coconut and palm oil—are also high in saturated fat.)

Cholesterol itself is not found in any plant food; it's made in the livers of animals, including humans. We make all we need. The cholesterol obtained from food is extra and accounts in part for the abnormally high blood cholesterol levels prevalent in this country. While numerous studies have associated elevated cholesterol levels with heart disease, a low blood cholesterol level may be a reasonable indicator of protection against other degenerative conditions as well.

"The higher the plasma cholesterol level, the higher is the risk for so-called diseases of affluence: cancers, heart disease, diabetes, the kinds of disease we see in the West," says T. Colin Campbell, Ph.D., a key researcher in the Cornell-Oxford Project on Nutrition, Health, and Environment, the largest population study of diet and health ever conducted. "This is pretty remarkable," says Dr. Campbell, "because the plasma cholesterol levels in China are roughly between 100 and 200 milligrams per deciliter. In other words, their high is our low. What this is really saying, in a sense, is that the lower the cholesterol level, the better. High cholesterol levels are related to the consumption of animal foods, and it apparently doesn't take very much of them." (Findings from the extensive study of Campbell and his team, what the *New York Times* called "the Grand Prix of epidemiology," are available in a highly readable book, *The China Study*.)

Even the so-called lean cuts of meat have significant levels of saturated fat plus cholesterol. Eating poultry is only a slight improvement and some fish can be extremely high in cholesterol, even though most fish is lower in fat content than meat. There are some vegetable foods that are high in fat—oils, nuts, seeds, olives, avocados, and, to a lesser degree, full-fat soybean products—but the fat in these foods is primarily unsaturated. These fats have not been implicated in heart disease as have the saturated fats prevalent in animal foods, but it's wise to avoid an excess of all fats. (Both saturated and unsaturated fats have the same high caloric density.)

Love-powered eating outshines the American diet in that the latter gives high-fat foods such as meat and eggs star billing at meals. Milk, eggs, butter, and cheese are also used in preparing other foods from side dishes to desserts, and high-fat vegetable foods, such as salad dressings, cooking oil, and peanut butter find their way into a conventional diet as well. A pure love-powered diet eliminates cholesterol and most saturated fat, so the majority of people can enjoy a moderate use of the richer plant foods without difficulty. Just use good judgment. For example, margarine, even that free of trans-fat, is never going to be a health food. Use such borderline items sparingly.

The SAD Is Deficient in Fiber

Meat and dairy products are devoid of the plant fiber required for normal peristaltic action of the colon. In addition, the refining of grains removes most of their fiber content. The upshot of all this is that difficulties in digestion and elimination are so common in "well-fed" societies that bran flakes, fiber-enriched breads, and natural fiber laxatives are common as well. But fiber shouldn't have to be added to the diet. It ought to be there already.

High-fiber diets help lower cholesterol by trapping bile acids in the intestinal tract and allowing them to be excreted, and such a diet is believed to protect against varicose veins, hemorrhoids, hiatus hernia, appendicitis, and gallstones, as well as constipation. The richest sources of fiber are whole grains and legumes; vegetables and fruits are fiber-filled as well.

The SAD Is Excessive in Protein

Periodically, "high-protein" becomes a buzzword for good nutrition, but we shouldn't be misled on this one. Protein is certainly necessary, but most Americans get far too much of it and that can be a problem. No more than fifteen percent of calories in a normal diet should come from protein, but Americans routinely eat animal foods that contain forty-one percent (skim milk, turkey), seventy-nine percent (cottage cheese), and even eighty-eight percent (water-packed tuna) protein.

Although you may have heard that protein burns fat, this assertion is based on the disease state of ketosis that occurs when you consume a risky diet of virtually only protein and fat, with no carbohydrate. In actuality, it's more likely that a high intake of protein—especially that from animal sources—may lead to overweight. In the China Health Study alluded to earlier, it was learned that the Chinese consumed, on average, twenty percent more calories per pound of body weight than Americans, but the Chinese were lighter and leaner by some twenty-five percent. Part of the reason for this is their level of physical exercise. (When I was in China, I saw bicycles carrying three adults and transporting pieces of furniture as if the bikes were two-wheeled moving vans.) But T. Colin Campbell believes that their low-protein intake (low in animal protein in particular) may play a part as well.

"It turns out that when one is on a low intake of animal protein, a higher proportion of the energy consumed is actually burned off as heat and it is not laid down as body fat," Dr. Campbell explains. "So a low-protein diet, which is characteristic of a vegetarian type of diet, allows obviously more energy to be consumed without running the risk of getting fat from that extra energy—those extra calories. This is an old observation, incidentally. It has been around for many, many years, although it has really been much ignored. It's clear that if you look at vegans (true vegetarians that eat only plant foods—no meats or dairy products) in this country, they tend to be rather lean. They tend not to have obesity problems."

Excess protein intake also causes the liver and kidneys to work harder, and it may increase the excretion of calcium and the occurrence of osteoporosis (see "Calcium or Cowcium?" later in this chapter).

Disease Prevention and the Vegetarian Edge

If I tell you that the proof of all this is in the pudding, you could tell me that I'm using a food addict's favorite phrase; but there's absolute truth in it. Following are some of the many ways in which vegetarians are generally better off than omnivores (meat-and-plant eaters).

Blood pressure. Studies repeatedly show that a low-fat vegetarian diet tends to produce lower blood pressure. This could be due to the trimness of vegetarians, but they also show markedly lower blood viscosity (thickness). The hormonal factors present in meat may also play a role. "Stress hormones are present in an animal at the time of slaughter. The same hormones that cause animals' blood pressure to rise cause ours to rise. It just takes a few molecules," explains George Eisman, R.D., author *A Basic Course in Vegetarian and Vegan Nutrition.*

Breast cancer. Women who eat meat daily (compared to those who eat it less than once a week) increase their risk of developing breast cancer by 3.8 times. Those who eat eggs daily (compared to once a week) increase their risk of breast cancer by 2.8 times. Factors accounting for this may include the way in which vegetarian women process estrogen, retaining less of it in their bodies than their meat-eating counterparts, and a statistically later onset of menses among younger vegan females.

Diabetes. The decreased chance of obesity in vegans puts them at lower risk for developing Type II (adult onset, although now showing up in children as well) diabetes. Further, according to *Reversing Diabetes* author Julian Whitaker, M.D., "A high-fat diet, even if it doesn't lead to obesity, may bring on diabetes in genetically predisposed individuals—perhaps because the cells of the body are so clogged with fat that they don't receive the insulin message to remove sugar from the bloodstream. The sugar (glucose) accumulates in the blood with disastrous results."

Low-fat diets high in unrefined carbohydrates have clinical application in treating diabetes. Administered under a physician's care, such diets frequently result in the elimination of medication (insulin or oral hypoglycemic agents) in adult-onset diabetes and a reduction in insulin as well as better general control for those with juvenile diabetes.

Heart disease. Vegans have very low cholesterol levels and a concurrently low incidence of heart disease. This finding is not new. Back in June 1961, an editorial in the *Journal of the American Medical Association* stated that a total vegetarian diet "could prevent 90 percent of our thromboembolic disease and 97 percent of our coronary occlusions." It was only in the late 1980s, however, that the work of Dean Ornish, M.D., and his colleagues at the University of California at San Francisco confirmed that coronary artery disease can be not only prevented but reversed with a low-fat, vegetarian diet in combination with lifestyle modification including exercise and stress-management techniques. Concurrent work at the Cleveland Clinic conducted by Caldwell Esselstyn, M.D., and extending out for twenty years, showed similar results with diet as the *only* factor.

Let Your Gourmet Come Out and Play

. . . .

If you think whole grains, vegetables, legumes, and fruits sound too basic for fine dining, read the following buffet brunch menu from a Physicians Committee for Responsible Medicine news conference. I'm not recommending seven-dessert spreads, and it's usually safest for food addicts to keep things simple. Nevertheless, a healthful, plant-based diet can dress up quite elegantly.

Menu

Creamy Banana-Date Shake
Chilled Melon Soup with Berries and
    Roasted Pine Nuts

Assorted Vegetable Lasagna
Tortellini in Pesto Sauce
Ratatouille Ravioli with Shallot Confit
Red Bell Pepper Sauce
Stuffed Grape Leaves with Rice and
    Almonds
Vegetarian Chili
Potato, Leek, and Tofu Tart
Orange Crème Brûlée
Lemon Trifle, Lemon Zest, and
    Strawberries
Piña Colada Mousse with Pineapple
Fruit Kebabs with Toasted Coconut
Apricot and Mango Sauce
Carrot Cake with Maple Syrup
Strawberry Shortcake

Obesity. Vegetarians who consume milk and eggs tend to be leaner than omnivores and vegans are even more so. Condensing evidence presented in a variety of academic journals, the EarthSave Foundation booklet *Our Food, Our Future* states that, compared to the general population with an obesity rate of 30.5 percent, only six percent of vegetarians are obese. Based on interviews with numerous physicians and other health care professionals who are intimately familiar with the vegan community, *Diet for a New America* author John Robbins estimates that the obesity rate of people eating a totally plant-based diet (like the one recommended in this book) is a mere two percent.

Osteoporosis. The brittle-bone disease that primarily affects postmenopausal women is less likely to occur among vegetarians because they do not have the high intake of protein that may cause calcium to be leached from the bones. Adequate but modest protein consumption combined with regular weight-bearing exercise appears to be the best defense against osteoporosis. Supplementary calcium has not been conclusively proven effective, and when extra calcium is taken in the form of dairy products, any possible benefit from the calcium may be offset by the additional protein in the milk or cheese. Several studies suggest that a diet high in fruits and vegetables may offer some protection. Curiously, the nations with the highest calcium intakes are the same ones with the highest osteoporosis rates.

Other diseases. Several cancers—including those of the ovaries, prostate, colon, and rectum—are statistically less common among vegetarians. Eliminating or drastically reducing meat consumption is standard in the treatment of gout (the purines in meat seem to be the aggravating factor here) and of impaired kidney function (in this case, intake of all high-protein foods is curtailed). Studies have shown vegetarians to have a decreased incidence of gallstones, kidney stones, diverticulosis (an intestinal disorder), and stroke. Stroke is the obstruction of an artery to the brain. When an artery to the heart is completely blocked, a heart attack occurs. The same condition—saturated fat and cholesterol impeding blood flow—can account for either. It's merely a matter of location. (Erectile dysfunction can result from similar blockages to the penis.)

Nutritionally Speaking

Prudence suggests that switching to a love-powered diet may well provide the best odds for a long, healthy, and enjoyable life. It would make sense that the same food program that protects against so many diseases and lacks so many of the components shown to be harmful to human health would also provide us with what we require nutritionally. According to the Dietary Guidelines for Americans, we should:

- Eat a variety of foods
- Maintain a healthy weight
- Choose a diet low in total fat, saturated fat, and cholesterol
- Choose a diet with plenty of vegetables, fruits, and grain products

- Use sugars only in moderation
- Use salt and sodium only in moderation
- Avoid alcoholic beverages or keep consumption moderate

A love-powered diet easily meets these recommendations.

The New Four Food Groups

Some twenty years ago, Physicians Committee for Responsible Medicine devised an easy dietary guideline for vegetarians called the "New Four Food Groups." While no longer new, they still work. We've alluded to these before. Here's a recap:

Whole grains. This group includes bread, pasta, hot or cold cereal, tortillas, and crackers, as long they're made from unrefined grains. Also in this group are grains such as corn, millet, barley, bulgur, buckwheat, and high-protein quinoa. Build meals around a hearty grain dish—grains are rich in fiber and other complex carbohydrates as well as protein, B vitamins, and zinc.

Fruit. Fruits are rich in fiber, vitamin C, and beta-carotene. Be sure to include at least one serving each day of fruits that are high in vitamin C—citrus fruits, melons, and strawberries are all good choices. Most of the time, choose whole fruit over fruit juices.

Vegetables. Vegetables are packed with nutrients; they provide vitamin C, beta-carotene, riboflavin, and other vitamins as well as iron, calcium, and fiber. Dark green leafy vegetables such as broccoli, collards, kale, mustard and turnip greens, romaine, and Swiss chard are especially good sources of these important nutrients. Dark yellow and orange vegetables such as carrots, winter squash, sweet potatoes, and pumpkin provide extra beta-carotene. Include generous portions of a variety of vegetables in your diet.

Legumes. Legumes—another name for beans, peas, and lentils—are all good sources of fiber, protein, iron, calcium, zinc, and B vitamins. Among the many members of this group are chickpeas (garbanzo beans), baked beans, soymilk, tofu, tempeh (a meaty fermented product that originated in Indonesia, and can be found in the freezer case at health food stores), texturized vegetable protein (TVP—sort of like Hamburger Helper but there won't be any hamburger), and peanuts. (Remember: peanuts and peanut butter are still high in fat.)

Round out your diet by regularly including a good source of vitamin B12, not reliably found in the foods from the plant kingdom. Most multivitamin/mineral supplements include this nutrient; enriched soy or rice-based milk substitutes and many cereals are also fortified with B12.

Food Group	Number of Servings	Serving Size
Whole Grains	four or more	half cup of hot cereal (i.e. oatmeal, cream of brown rice) one oz. of dry cereal (i.e. shredded wheat, Uncle Sam, NutriGrain, or other cold cereal made with whole grain) one slice of bread (whole-wheat, rye or spelt)
Fruits	two or more	one medium piece of fruit half cup of cooked fruit half cup of fruit juice
Vegetables	five or more	one cup of raw vegetables half cup of cooked vegetables
Legumes	two or three	half cup of cooked beans four oz. of tofu or tempeh eight oz. of fortified soymilk

Sometimes having a simple list like the one above is helpful, especially if you're feeling unsure of taking what seems like a major leap. Use these serving numbers to help you plan healthy meals, but don't get caught in a diet-like trap. These are guidelines. Rest assured—natural foods are nutritious foods. If you eat a variety of them, you'll not ordinarily have to weigh, measure, or count servings.

It's gratifying to see knowledgeable professionals formulate nutritional guidelines that are ideal for both human and planetary health. Even without a system of food groups, however, it's not difficult to plan an adequate diet from natural vegetarian foods. Nature has designed these to meet our needs, not just adequately but abundantly. Of course, some planning is required, particularly because low-fat vegetarian foods aren't yet the major menu items at fast-food restaurants and roadside diners, which often seem the most convenient places to stop. Your choice of restaurants will gradually change as your style of eating changes, and you may find that you like your own cooking more and more.

In spite of abundant information to the contrary, many people fear that in making the transition to simpler eating, they will miss out on specific nutrients, including protein, iron, calcium, riboflavin, and vitamin B12. Here's a look at each and how to ensure that you'll get enough.

Protein Again

We've talked about getting too much, so now let's talk about getting enough. Legumes, whole grains, soy foods, some nuts and seeds (notably hemp seeds), and even dark leafy greens are surprisingly rich in protein. In fact, if you could design a diet built around natural starches and vegetables that provided enough calories to maintain normal weight but was deficient in protein, you'd be famous because no one has been able to do so yet. The only way a person on a natural-foods, animal-free diet could become deficient in protein would be to take in too few calories due to excessive fasting or dieting, or by living *solely* on those few fruits that have less than five percent of calories as protein.

But what about amino acids, those building blocks of protein that some people believe total vegetarians can only obtain by eating grains, legumes, and nuts in precise mathematical combinations? You can save your calculator for doing your taxes: you won't need it to prepare your dinner. Eat a variety of natural foods over the course of the day and protein complementing will take care of itself. "In fact," says registered dietician George Eisman, "all plant proteins are complete. Some are higher in certain amino acids than others, but by eating enough of any

The Raw Alternative

. . . .

The latest twist on plant-based eating to catch the attention of popular culture is the raw, or living-food, lifestyle. This entails making up seventy-five percent or more of the diet from uncooked fruits, vegetables, sprouts, nuts, and seeds. Those who are attracted to what may seem like an extreme dietary choice find it a revitalizing manner of eating and living. Although many people "go raw" as a means of healing some disorder, the first benefit most notice is weight loss, usually a lot of it quickly. One reason for this is that a raw diet is very low in sodium so the new raw-fooder loses a lot of water weight, but this way of eating is also naturally low in calories and the metabolism seems to love using these light, pure foods for body processes rather than fat storage.

Raw-fooders also report that they experience increased energy, a clearer complexion, and better sleep, often needing less sleep than before. Those who do eat some cooked food find that something like steamed broccoli, brown rice, or a baked potato is a change-of-pace treat, so they have no desire for the sweets, chips, or fries that were so enticing when broccoli and brown rice was the "healthy food."

The raw philosophy is, simply stated, that of all animal life, only humans apply heat to our food; the prevalence of disease throughout our history and at the present time may have an intimate connection to breaking what raw-fooders see as an obvious law of nature. Not only does cooking decrease the available nutrient content of many foods, heating any food over 118 degrees kills the enzymes present in it. Enzymes are catalysts required for myriad physiological processes, including the digestion and metabolism of everything we eat. When we consume cooked foods, we draw on our own finite enzyme stores. With raw foods and their full enzyme complement, energy soars because we're getting abundant nourishment and not robbing the dwindling supply of enzymes we were born with.

There's a metaphysical side to raw food as well, the idea that *life force*, what the yogis call *prana* and Chinese medicine and martial arts refer to as *chi*, is what we really live on. Breathing pure air, drinking pure water, enjoying good companionship, and doing spiritual practice all increase the *prana* to which we have access. So does eating unheated, unprocessed food with its own life force intact.

The "food groups" for a raw vegan diet are a little different: vegetables (including sprouts and freshly extracted vegetable juices, with an emphasis on protein-and-nutrient-rich dark leafy greens); fruits (fresh and dried—the dried fruits are

The Raw Alternative (continued)

. . . .

usually soaked a few hours before eating to awaken their life force); and nuts and seeds (again, these are usually soaked to deactivate the enzyme-inhibitors present in dry nuts and seeds; soaking also lowers the fat content since some of that caloric energy is used to begin the sprouting process that soaking incites).

Because vegetables are so low in calories, raw-fooders need to eat enough fruit to get adequate calories so that they don't depend too much on the higher-fat foods. However, people who eat this way seem to be able to get by with consuming somewhat more fat than the conventional recommendations, probably because the unheated oils they consume (mostly in the form of nuts, seeds, and avocado) are more efficiently used by the body than heated fats are.

Raw food-eating has become a fascinating subculture with its own experts and celebrities. One of these is Philip McCluskey (www.lovingraw.com) who slimmed from four hundred pounds to half that, in a two-year period. "Most people find that excess weight comes off effortlessly after going to a raw vegan diet," says McCluskey. "By switching to a simple, live food diet, not only does your weight regulate, but often there's a drastic improvement in your energy, happiness, and overall quality of life."

I myself have taken to the high-raw lifestyle in the past year and although I don't care to make it a religion or go a hundred percent raw, I must say that I feel younger, lighter, and more alive than I have in years. It may be that eating raw foods is the Lamborghini of my midlife crisis, but I feel too good to give it up now.

There are several raw-food resources in the appendices. If you'd like a head start, take a look at one of my favorite cookless books for beginners, Jennifer Cornbleet's *Raw Food Made Easy for 1 or 2 People.* There's also a companion DVD so you can see how simple this kind of food prep can be.

one plant protein, all needs can be adequately met. The irony is that an incomplete protein does exist: it's gelatin, an animal derivative." (There's more on protein in "Nutshell Nutrition: The Macronutrients," one of the appendices at the back of this book.)

The Popeye Principle

Natural foods from the plant kingdom make a respectable showing in terms of iron. Dried fruits (prunes, raisins, apricots, and peaches), dried beans and lentils, whole grains such as rye and wheat, and green leafy vegetables are all rich in this mineral. It has long been held, however, that iron from animal sources (heme iron) is more readily assimilated than non-heme iron from plants. Also, phytates (a form of phytic acid) present in whole grains have been believed to detrimentally inhibit iron utilization, although this has never been shown to cause iron deficiency in humans.

"In research, the focus is often on single or isolated nutrients or other substances," says Suzanne Havala Hobbs, Dr.P.H., M.S., R.D., who has done research into the iron sufficiency of vegetarian diets, based in large part on the China Study. "Results often ignore the reality of the complex nutrient interactions that occur within the context of the total diet. In this case, plant components such as fiber and phytates apparently do not have a significant effect on iron absorption in vegetarian diets that contain adequate vitamin C from fruits and vegetables. Vegetarians in the United States tend to have good iron status."

Just as iron absorption can be impeded, it can also be enhanced. One way to do this is to eat one or more foods rich in vitamin C, such as citrus fruit, tomatoes, or green peppers, along with an iron-rich food. Another way to add iron to your diet is to use cast-iron cookware. "It was found that a 100-gram serving of spaghetti sauce prepared in iron cookware contained 87.5 milligrams of iron compared to only 3 when cooked in a glass vessel," reports Agatha Thrash, M.D., in *Nutrition for Vegetarians.*

It's also possible to overdo on iron. This may pose an increased risk of heart disease in men and postmenopausal women. This is why multivitamin/mineral supplements geared to those of middle age and beyond (the "silver" formulas) contain little or no iron.

Calcium or Cowcium?

Perhaps even more ubiquitous than the myth that meat is necessary for protein is the myth that cow's milk is necessary for calcium. This defies logic in several ways.

First of all, over half of the world's population, primarily those of African and Asian descent, lack the enzyme to digest cow's milk. Just because enzyme tablets or liquid can be taken to compensate for this doesn't make it a disease or abnormality.

On the contrary, the ability to tolerate dairy foods may in fact be an adaptation to their consumption rather than an indication of normal digestive capacity. It is, after all, *only the human species that drinks milk after weaning or takes the milk of another animal.* (You may want to stop for a second and let that one sink in. It's an astonishing fact the first time you think of it.) All the calcium in cow's milk comes from the grass and grain eaten by the cow. Although you may not choose to refrain from consuming dairy products, it's important for you to know that humans, as well as cows, can get all the calcium we need from plant foods.

In fact, virtually any vegetable food you might choose has some calcium in it. In his book *Vegan Nutrition: Pure and Simple,* Dr. Michael Klaper lists these calcium all-stars: collards, kale, oats, chickpeas, trail mix made of one part almonds to two parts raisins, and calcium-fortified tofu. (Tofu made with calcium sulfate will say so on the label.) Calcium-fortified and enriched versions of soymilk and rice milk— tasty substitutes for cow's milk, available at health food stores and some supermarkets—are also easy ways to boost calcium intake.

Moreover, the total amount of calcium that you'll need on a vegetarian diet is probably lower than you think. This is because the high protein content of a meat-based diet is likely to cause calcium to be withdrawn from the bones. To eliminate the breakdown products of excess protein, the kidneys are forced to work overtime excreting more urine. And minerals—notably calcium—are in that urine.

In researching this information, I was astonished to learn that, as noted above, the countries with the highest consumption of dairy products also have the highest rates of osteoporosis. This isn't so amazing when you realize that those are also the nations with high protein intakes. Animal protein may be more of a culprit in this regard than an equal amount of vegetable protein. In a study done at the University of Texas Southwestern Medical Center in Dallas, people who switched from a vegetarian diet to one containing eggs, red meat, poultry, and fish excreted more calcium, *although the actual amount of protein ingested remained the same.* The high sulfur content of animal protein is thought to be the cause. In the body, sulfur turns into the acid sulfate, which must be buffered. To do this, calcium and other minerals are withdrawn from the bones.

Although the Daily Value for calcium is a thousand milligrams, the World Health Organization recommends only five hundred milligrams daily. A total vegetarian diet—unless you make a point of eating high-calcium foods every day—will probably provide less calcium than one containing dairy products, but it will also be free of excess protein and thus help to ensure a positive calcium balance within your body.

Writing in *Nutrition Health Review,* Robert Kradjian, M.D., sheds some light on this complex issue: "We [Americans] are increasing the calcium recommendation and experiencing an increasing incidence of osteoporosis while other women in the world are doing well on little as 200 milligrams a day. The problem is that you simply can't force oral calcium into bones. . . . It is the calcium balance, not the calcium intake, that counts. . . . If more calcium is being lost from the body than enters it, there will exist a negative balance, and osteoporosis will eventually result."

Riboflavin

Most Americans get riboflavin (vitamin B2) in dairy products, meat (especially liver), and eggs, so some nutritionists have expressed concern that vegetarians will lack this vitamin. This is on par with telling someone who's chauffeured to the office by limousine that she's missing out by not driving herself like most Americans. In fact, riboflavin is found abundantly in leafy greens, legumes, and nutritional yeast, and to a lesser but still significant extent in whole grains. Avoiding empty-calorie junk foods that displace nutritious foods in the diet is the best way to ensure adequate riboflavin intake.

Vitamin B12

Vitamin B12 is a fascinating nutrient about which more is probably unknown than known. But we do have the following facts.

- Vitamin B12 is an essential nutrient—without it, severe neurological damage can occur.
- Only a minuscule amount is needed—six micrograms a day.
- In almost every case of reported B12 deficiency disease, the cause was not a dietary shortfall but the patient's lack of *intrinsic factor,* a substance produced in the body that's necessary for the absorption of this vitamin.
- Vitamin B12 is made by microorganisms and therefore is not known to occur naturally in foods of plant origin that have been scrubbed clean.
- It's stored in the body for long periods—three to eight years. After three years (or immediately in the case of children, pregnant women, and nursing mothers), total vegetarians need to include in their diets a supplementary source of vitamin B12.

Beyond this, there are many unanswered questions. Numerous vegans who have been observed over the past sixty years have not taken supplemental B12 and, almost without exception, they've done just fine. Probably the tiny amounts of B12 needed were supplied by the microbes living in their mouths and intestinal tracts. Nevertheless, total vegetarians are advised to include a reliable source of biologically available vitamin B12 in their diets to meet the Daily Value. This usually means taking a tablet about once a week since the daily requirement is so small. B12 is apparently better absorbed when taken on its own rather than as part of a multivitamin/mineral supplement.

The Daily Value can also be met with regular intake of foods fortified with this vitamin, including fortified soy or rice milk and many of the breakfast cereals at the supermarket. Certain fermented foods such as raw sauerkraut and the Chinese probiotic drink *Kombucha* (www.gtskombucha.com) also have enough of this nutrient to be able to list it on their labels.

One More Thing

A few new vegans, especially those who jump enthusiastically into raw foods (see "The Raw Alternative" on page 119), actually have to make an effort to get enough calories. You may be thinking, "I could use more problems like that," but if you do find that you're losing weight too rapidly or losing more than you set out to, you may need to increase your portions.

You'll be eating more food on a low-fat, natural foods program than with any other approach you've taken to lose weight or maintain the weight that's right for you. The caloric equivalent of a four-ounce hamburger and twelve measly fries is two cups of brown rice, topped with one cup of cabbage, one cup of cauliflower, one cup of mushrooms, and half an onion stir-fried with nearly a tablespoon of olive oil. Since oil is the most calorific food, steaming those vegetables instead of sautéing them means that you could double their amount or have a wheat roll on the side.

Of course, you don't have to be concerned with juggling calories any longer. You'll eat, you'll finish, and then you'll follow your heart to some noble pursuit or great adventure. (Or maybe you'll just wash the dishes, but you won't have to think about food while you're doing it.) Should you need extra calories to maintain normal weight, increase your amounts of the more concentrated foods like bread and pasta, and (unless you have a medical contraindication to this) you can be more liberal in your use of the "rich relatives"—concentrated sweets like dates and dried fruits and oil-rich whole foods such as nuts, nut butters (almonds, pecans, cashews, and macadamias make delicious butters), olives, and avocados.

Vitamin YOU

Foods contain nutrients, but *you*, with your unique physical self and the mind that so influences your body, are the nutrient processor. You're nourished not by what's on your plate but by what you can assimilate into your body. Nutrient antagonists abound in most modern lives. Excess stress can create a need for more B-complex vitamins. Diuretics can deplete potassium supply. A sedentary lifestyle and the use of caffeine, alcohol, cigarettes, birth control pills, certain antibiotics, and even aspirin can drain vitamin and mineral reserves. It is therefore obvious that your entire way of life affects your nutritional status.

Part of the beauty of love-powered living is that it's not primarily about what you eat. The changes in the foods you choose come about as a result of changes in your consciousness, in your awareness, and in your willingness to love yourself and others. When you no longer need to eat for a fix because of the quiet miracle happening to you mentally and spiritually, this new way of eating can outwardly express your inner transformation. Ultimately, the most important nutritional element is vitamin YOU. It's activated by contact with a Higher Power, supportive friends, an appreciation of life and every creature that has it, and supplementary doses of gratitude and wonder.

CHAPTER EIGHT

FOOD FOR LIFE

I'm going to be pragmatic now and deal with grocery carts, restaurant menus, and the culinary basics of a love-powered way of nourishing ourselves. While eating *destructively* has been the problem, eating *constructively* is an essential part of solving it. For this reason, we need to talk about food.

If you're a food addict, be sure that you feel ready to read and think about food right now. As long as you are in the state of spiritual fitness that *Alcoholics Anonymous* refers to as "a position of neutrality, safe and protected," you can open yourself without fear to all the useful information you'll need. You're not fraternizing with the enemy by learning a better way of eating and new cooking techniques— you are instead developing a helpful and healthy relationship with food.

We're going to be viewing this from a perspective that may be unlike any you've taken before. Knowing how a food tastes and its nutrient profile has its place. Recognizing how we feel about certain foods is equally important.

Take, for example, string beans. If you're going to use the fresh ones, they need to have their ends removed. It's tedious but I'm convinced that such chores are far more meaningful than they appear because they speak of our connection with nature—a connection that is stabilizing and healing.

Of course it's easier to open a bag of frozen beans. They don't have any more calories than fresh ones, and nutritionally they're virtually identical. Sometimes saving minutes can be a legitimate priority. The price paid for the convenience, however, is that we give up the tactile and participatory experience of taking the fresh option. We tend to think that a good cardio workout is the only activity that helps keep a body fit and trim. That's not so. Snapping beans and shelling peas will do it, too, just in a different way. Activities such as these give us a psychic kinship with the foods we eat, with the soil, the seasons—the source of physical life and nourishment. Binge eating is in direct opposition to this kinship, because it shuts us off from life.

A Gentle Transition

You'll soon experience a great many changes—changes in your outlook toward food as well as in what and how you eat. Before we look at the dietary aspects, let's work a little with change itself. To do this, it will help to make some lists.

First, jot down three really important positive changes that you've made in your life, actions that in retrospect you're glad you took. Now, think back to when each was just beginning. How was it? Did you love whatever it was without reservation or was there a period of adjustment? Was your positive change (going off to college, moving to another state or country, making a midlife career move) comfortable from the start, or did you have to get used to it?

My list of important positive things includes (1) living in London after I graduated from high school, (2) becoming a parent, and (3) giving up my regular magazine job to freelance full-time. These are among the red-letter events of my life, turning points for which I'm deeply grateful. Nevertheless, when I arrived alone in the huge capital of a foreign country at the age of eighteen, I wanted to turn around and run back through customs in the other direction. When my daughter was born, I realized that not one of the dozens of books I'd read about pregnancy and birth had prepared me for the reality of caring for a tiny human being. And once I left the security of a steady job for the sink-or-swim uncertainty of self-employment, I felt that I'd joined a trapeze act that didn't use a net.

These separate and qualitatively different events took place over a twenty-year time span, yet each required patience and persistence from me for its richness and beauty to become apparent. You've no doubt noticed this during the important positive events in your own life. Now you're about to chalk up another. The change for you in terms of diet could be relatively minor (maybe you're already a vegetarian but you're still attached to hefty quantities of pizza or yogurt) or it may call for a ninety-degree turnaround in your eating habits. Whether subtle or startling in its particulars, this change will be significant. Allow yourself a gentle transition.

If choosing to eat in a way that expresses love to yourself and others is a commitment that grows from your deepest self, you'll realize that you're in this for the duration. You don't have to know everything right away. You only need to choose the very best foods you know of for today's three meals. Tomorrow, you'll know a little more and your choices then will reflect that.

I'd like to help you ease into this transition by reminding you of the love-powered eating with which you're already familiar. There are times in your life, probably many such times, when you aren't eating for a fix—when you eat some fresh, natural food and really enjoy it. You already know how to do this; you'll just be doing it more. Let's start with exploring the basic food groups of a plant-based diet—fruits, vegetables, whole grains, and legumes—in a gustatory way.

Fruit—Nature's Candy Store

Chances are, you eat fruit now and you probably like it. Nearly everybody does. It's possible to become so jaded by overindulgence in refined sweets (candy, pastries, and the like) that the delicate flavors of fruit are no longer appealing. After a few days away from sugary foods, though, fruit becomes a real treat. It's sweet and delicious, a veritable vitamin factory, and virtually fat-free. Fruit makes an ideal breakfast, a handy snack, or a light dessert that's always ready. You don't have to do anything to it, just enjoy.

Write down your ten favorite fruits. That sounds like quite a few, but it won't be hard once you get started. Think of the exotic fruits you had on your trip to Hawaii. Remember that interesting melon you found at the greengrocer's last summer, and the wild strawberries you picked in your grandmother's yard so long ago. You'll find that you already know some of nature's tastiest tidbits—and there are lots more where those came from. Now allow me to introduce you to my ten favorites.

Bananas. Most people aren't aware that there are more than a dozen varieties of banana, each distinct. In northern climates, our selection isn't terrific (a banana is a banana), but even these make my list because, when frozen, they turn a simple blender drink into something frothy and luscious. They can even become a treat that's astonishingly like ice cream. Use really ripe bananas (the skins need to be well flecked with brown), peel them, and then freeze them in airtight containers. Then chop the bananas into one-inch rounds and purée them in your food processor using the metal "S" blade. You'll need to scrape down the sides with a spatula every so often until the banana is processed into a delectable "soft-serve."

Cantaloupe. Cantaloupe probably wouldn't make my top ten list if it weren't for the smooth and tasty shakes that can be made from the juicy, ripe ones. Chop a cantaloupe into cubes and put these in a blender with the smallest amount of water necessary to get the blender to liquefy the fruit. It's really amazing how thick and creamy this turns out—an exquisite light breakfast or summertime cooler.

Cherries. Cherries remind me of my father, of visiting home and going with him to a certain produce merchant at the city market for the darkest, sweetest Bing cherries in season. Because of their pits, cherries can't be bolted down. It seems to me like nature's way of saying, "I put a lot into these, so slow down and relish them."

Dates. Fresh dates are sweet treats from nature but difficult to find, so when we think of dates in this country, we're usually talking about the dried ones. This makes them too rich to eat as a snack except for active children, athletes, and people trying to gain weight, but four or five big Medjool dates with lettuce leaves, peanut butter-stuffed celery, and a crunchy Rome Beauty apple or two make my favorite autumn lunch. (*Caveat: some compulsive eaters find dates too much like candy to keep around the house. If this or any food causes you more angst than pleasure, avoid it and choose from the abundance that's still available to you.*)

Mangoes. These are best when very ripe. You can often get them on sale when they look past their prime but are really just right for eating. Make a crosscut into the fruit starting on top and going one-quarter of the way down the sides. You can peel a mango by hand from there. Have plenty of napkins nearby. Mangoes are juicy, messy, and delectable. (A peeled, ripe frozen mango can be put through a good quality juicer for a heavenly sorbet.)

Papayas. Papaya is an acquired taste, and it's true that most of those shipped north can't compare with the tree-ripened tropical gems. Still, if you let one completely ripen until it's yellow and spotted and has the same give as a ready avocado, it can be a real delight. (Don't eat the black seeds that you'll scoop from the center; they're bitter.)

Peaches. Peaches let me know it's summer. When there's a little "give" in response to a gentle squeeze, these seasonal delights are ready to enjoy. For "peaches and cream," I slice the fruit and top it with a little soy creamer (found in natural food stores). Alternatively, I make a luscious cashew cream by blending raw cashews half and half with water, sweetening with a little agave nectar, and straining through a mesh bag. (Raw cashews are sold natural food stores. Buying from the bulk bins saves money. And when you're going to be blending them anyway, choose raw cashew pieces rather than whole nuts for even more savings.)

Persimmons. Life is too short to consider persimmons too expensive. I'd never tasted this fruit until I was thirty years old and visited a resort in south Texas where custard-like persimmons were lunchtime specialties. I still get them often in late fall and winter, and although they do cost more than less exotic fruits, I think the persimmons and I are both worth it. (Eat them when they are very soft. When you think they're ripe, give them another couple of days.)

Raspberries. I love how these fragile, fragrant berries taste. I can remember getting a half-pint from a roadside stand in Indiana on a road trip once and savoring every berry right there by the side of the highway. That's when I realized that this slow savoring was the exact opposite of binge eating. I have Indiana raspberries to thank for the insight.

Watermelon. Watermelon is an air conditioner that you eat. I never liked it much until I learned the secret of watermelon connoisseurship: Eat it by itself, not with other foods. Its exquisite juiciness can't be appreciated in the company of other foods. (And people who have trouble digesting melon often find that eating it alone remedies that problem.) A terrific watermelon will be heavy—that's the sweet juice weighing in.

There are also, of course, apples, oranges, grapefruit, tangerines, starfruit, honeydew, pomegranates, pineapples, kumquats, pears (and prickly pears!), nectarines, apricots, grapes, kiwifruit, figs, plums, blueberries, blackberries, and more. There are fruits for every climate and all times of year. You can see already that nature is not miserly—and we've only discussed one of the many tasty offerings from her pantry. Here are some tips.

- *Remember that fruit can be a quick breakfast, the perfect snack, or a de-light-ful dessert.* (If eating fruit on top of other food doesn't agree with you, save your dessert for a couple of hours after the meal.)
- *Eat fruit when it's fully ripe.* Much fruit is picked green for shipping and, with the exception of citrus and apples, often needs to ripen after you get it home. Bananas ripen best in a brown paper bag, and placing a banana in such a bag with unripe papayas, avocados, or pears hastens their ripening as well.
- *Wash dirt, surface chemicals, and waxes from fruit (and vegetables) with a diluted detergent mixture, then rinse well.* Or use a special cleaning product that's available for this purpose at health food stores. If produce is heavily waxed, you're better off peeling it.
- *Eat whole fruits most of the time instead of drinking fruit juice.* Because the fiber has been removed, the natural sugars in fruit juice can enter your bloodstream very quickly. Using some apple or pineapple in a green juice is fine, though, since the green veggies cut the sugar.
- *When you do drink fruit juice, dilute it by half with water.* Sparkling water and juice over ice make a refreshing soda. Sip juice slowly, and prepare it fresh whenever possible. Citrus juicers, manual and electric, are inexpensive and easy to find in department and culinary stores. (A more elaborate juicer that juices all fruits and vegetables is a good investment, too. The Jack LaLanne Power Juicer is reliable and very affordable; Breville juicers are sturdy, versatile, and easy to use and clean; and the Green Star is an investment-quality professional juicer for the aficionado.)
- *Other than for the occasional special dish, eat fruit that's fresh and uncooked.* Frozen unsweetened berries and mixed fruit may be used in smoothies (blended fruit drinks) or when fresh fruit is not available. Use canned fruit, even the juice-packed kind, only as a last resort. All canned foods have been heated.

- *Because they're very sweet, treat dates and dried fruits as delicacies.* If you wish to release weight, have these only in moderation: no more than half a dozen dates, figs, or prunes or a handful of raisins a couple of times a week. Dried fruit is best soaked—reconstituted with water to more clearly resemble its fresh state—or save these rich foods for use in other dishes—to sweeten hot cereal or garnish a salad, for instance, or to add to breads and muffins.
- *Plant a fruit tree.* Plant two. Plant ten. Some kind of fruit tree will grow almost anywhere. Start with a dwarf tree that will mature rapidly so you'll have something to pick without a long wait. Something momentous happens when you get fruit from a tree you've planted. You deserve that experience and the Earth needs every oxygen-producing tree it can get.

Everything's Coming Up Veggies

Many adults are still stuck in the six-year-old's notion that vegetables are "yucky." Vegetables carry the stigma in many people's minds of being "rabbit food"—dietetic stand-ins for something they'd rather eat. "I can eat ten carrots when I'm on a diet," I was once told, "but when I'm not on a diet, I don't touch a carrot." Despite these tainted views, vegetables—leafy greens, in particular—are nutritional powerhouses, and according to the Center for Science in the Public Interest, you can't go wrong with any vegetable (unless you fry it).

Let's face it: it takes some sophistication to appreciate vegetables. Children don't have it. The unimaginative who think of vegetables as canned peas and the lettuce on a burger don't have it either. But you do and we're going to explore that now. Think of a vegetable you honestly like. It needs to be one that you enjoy without cream sauce, gobs of butter, or deep-frying. What's the vegetable you enjoy raw or steamed until it's bright and crisp? Write it down.

My favorite vegetable is broccoli. When I used to fast, I didn't crave the chips and candy bars that had gotten me in trouble, but I dreamed of broccoli—lightly steamed with a squeeze of fresh lemon. Even then, my subconscious knew the good stuff. Nowadays, I fix broccoli at least twice a week and order steamed broccoli with garlic sauce on the side every time I go to a Chinese restaurant. My body seems to purr when it's had broccoli.

How often do you eat your favorite vegetable? Is it one that can be enjoyed both cooked and raw? Have you tried it both ways? Let's start a new list. Write down ten other vegetables you like. Make two columns: one of five vegetables you like raw and one of five you like cooked. (Some could be listed in both columns, but be sure to put down ten different vegetables altogether.) Here are mine:

Favorite Home-Cooked Vegetables

1. *Asparagus* is a marvelous luxury. Try it slightly steamed with a touch of herbal seasoning such as Mrs. Dash.
2. *Fresh peas.* I eat them right from the pod, quickly steamed.
3. *Chinese wood ear mushrooms.* Chewy and hearty, wood ears have a consistency that helps some people get over a yearning for meat. I like them scored with crosscuts on top and sautéed in a little oil and sherry with a dash of lemon juice and a few snips of parsley. They can also be boiled for a minute and used in other vegetable or grain dishes, soups, or stir-fries.
4. *Spaghetti squash.* This big, oval yellow squash is lots of fun since its meat, when cooked, is like strings of spaghetti. Scoop the seeds from a halved squash, cut into quarters, and steam, or prick the skin and bake it whole. Serve with an herbal seasoning and plenty of garlic, or with fresh tomato sauce.
5. *Kale.* Not only does kale pack in calcium, iron, and vitamin A, but it can be delicious, too. Dark leafy greens have the reputation of being strong and bitter (maybe that's why salad bars often have kale around the bowls for garnish instead of in them for eating). Greens don't need to be intimidating, though.

    Versatile kale can be chopped or shredded (I use kitchen shears for this). Remove the tough stems; steam the leaves in a vegetable steamer for five to six minutes, and season with a little lemon juice, ground black pepper and, optionally, olive oil and salt. You can enjoy this super-green as a salad, too, if you chop it finely; massage in a dressing of lemon juice, cider vinegar, and olive oil; season as you like and marinate overnight. Kale is also a terrific addition to a green drink. The wake-up beverage that gets me through an hour at the gym is juice made from one head of romaine, four or five sprigs of kale, one lemon, and two apples—yum.

Favorite Sun-cooked (i.e., Raw) Vegetables

1. *Arugula.* This is no wimpy vegetable but a Mediterranean contribution to a super salad that makes its presence known. Its taste can vary—sometimes in summer becoming quite hot and spicy—giving a gourmet touch to any season's salad. Clean it well and use sparingly until you become an arugula devotee.

2. *Carrots.* I go through a peeler at least once a year because our household carrot consumption rivals that of Peter Rabbit's. I like eating carrots whole (the miniature ones are great for munching) but I'm also apt to shred a couple in the food processor and use carrot instead of lettuce or sprouts on a sandwich.

   Carrot-raisin salad is another favorite at our house. You don't need mayonnaise for this—just mix shredded carrots with raisins and toss with a little pineapple juice and, if you like, a handful of sunflower seeds. If you like the mayo texture and flavor, the vegan alternatives such *Nayonaise* and *Vegenaise*, at natural food stores, are dead ringers for the real stuff.

   I'm a fan of carrot juice as well. Like fruit juices, it's sweet and lacks fiber, but it's packed with beta-carotene and energizing enzymes. Carrot juice is also the tasty base for making blends with less-sweet vegetable juices. Carrot/beet and carrot/celery/parsley juices are wonderful. When I drink them, I feel as if I'm doing something really special for myself. Make fresh and sip slowly. A stemmed goblet doesn't hurt either.

3. *Fresh corn, cut from the cob.* When it's harvest time for corn and you can get it straight from someone's garden or just picked at a farmers' market, young corn is sweet and juicy and perks up a salad quite nicely. (Baking corn on the cob is another good idea. The result is a much more flavorful vegetable than when it's boiled. It also roasts beautifully over a fire or in coals on a picnic or camping trip.)

4. *Sweet red peppers.* Sweet red peppers usually cost a little more than their more prominent green brethren (green because they're not really ripe yet), but the taste and additional nutrients make up for the added cost. Red bell pepper is also so pretty. A rainbow salad of bright green spinach, a few shreds of purple cab-

bage, and bright red rings of sweet pepper feeds your eyes before you even pick up a fork.

5. *Cauliflower.* This is my favorite of crudités. So unlike the overcooked, grayish mush that passed for cauliflower in the school cafeteria, raw cauliflower is tasty without being strident, and has a dandy crunch.

Raw vegetables must be fresh in order to be palatable. I'll admit to having cooked sagging spinach, yellowing broccoli, and limp carrots when I wouldn't have served them as a salad or crudités. You've probably done the same thing. There's nothing wrong with "waste not, want not," but it goes to show that vegetables that are delicious raw are the cream of the crop.

Now we each have lists of our ten favorite vegetables to include in salads, on relish trays, as steamed side dishes, or in casseroles and stir-fries. Starchy vegetables like potatoes, yams, and winter squash have enough substance to be entrées on their own. Following a salad with a steamed vegetable platter served with rolls or rice is a lovely meal, particularly in late summer when garden vegetables are most abundant. A salad itself can be a main dish when a heavier food like pasta, brown rice, or chickpeas is included in it; and hot vegetable soup with your own cornbread or bran muffins makes a fine winter lunch or late supper.

If your thumb has the slightest hint of green, consider doing a little gardening or becoming a regular farmers' market shopper. Get the freshest-looking produce you can find and afford. Stay away from canned vegetables: They are overcooked before they ever see your stove, and most are heavily salted. Experiment with vegetables. For each one you're not so fond of, there will be two or more that become your perennial favorites. Choose vegetables for their colors, textures, nuances of flavor. And don't forget the joy of snapping beans.

Grains Whole and Hearty

Grains are the foods that let you know that you ate. Whole grains are especially satisfying because they're substantial. You have to chew them. And when you chew grains, the digestive process starts right there in your mouth. The starches break down into their component sugars and the whole-wheat bread or brown rice you're eating tastes heavenly.

If you've always eaten refined grains like white rice and white-flour products, the natural grains may at first seem tough or coarsely textured. Don't feel that you have to change overnight to all whole grains. There will probably always be times at restaurants or in social situations when only refined grains are available. Unless the particular food is a binge provoker for you, it's OK. You're improving your diet, not engaging in an endurance trial.

Give yourself some credit. Maybe you already eat oatmeal every morning and you truly prefer whole-wheat bread, but you can't stand the thought of brown spaghetti. You're already ahead of the game. Give yourself some time. It won't be long before most of the refined stuff will taste like puffed air. Once you think of grains as generally referring to the whole grains that give an appetite what it came for and then send it on its way, it'll be much easier for you to see grains as a main course.

Let's go back to the list. Write down three meals you like that have a grain entrée. You can include pasta, waffles or pancakes, a rice dish, fresh bread with soup, or even a special sandwich. Write it down even if the way you eat it now is high in fat or contains animal ingredients. For example, you're probably used to pancakes made with milk and eggs. You can, however, make great pancakes that contain neither and use whole-wheat flour, too. Even pizza can be considered a grain-based entrée if it has a really good crust, is topped with sauce and vegetables, and substitutes a nice vegan mozzarella for the cheese.

There's probably a lot more variety in the grains available than you may think. In addition to the familiar ones like wheat, rice, oats, and corn, there are many unusual varieties, mostly found in stores that sell natural or gourmet foods. Experiment with an uncommon grain. Sometimes trying something new is a good exercise in risk-taking. Ruts have a way of making themselves deeper, and the same-old-food rut is one of the easiest to get out of. So make millet or kasha or quinoa for dinner. It will probably be a tremendous success. And what if it isn't? Peanut butter sandwiches are great when a new recipe bombs.

Keep the following grain facts in mind.

You don't have to skimp on your portions. You won't be eating gluttonously, but you'll be able to have ample, restaurant-size servings of pasta, enough rice to fill you up, and sandwiches that needn't be open-faced.

The old proscription against eating two starches at a meal no longer applies. You may not want both rice and potatoes or oatmeal and toast, but with this way of eating there's nothing to stop you from having them.

Promote grains from side dish to main course in both your thinking and your meals. (Remember that starchy vegetables like potatoes, yams, and winter squash as well as the low-fat, high-carbohydrate chestnut all have entrée potential.)

Start the switch from refined to whole grains by re-visualizing them. When someone says "bread," for example, consciously replace white with whole wheat in your mental image.

If you're afraid of grains (you think that they're fattening or you've often binged on baked goods), be clear on the tremendous difference between solid, sustaining whole grains and empty carbohydrates like pale, lifeless breads and cakes, and the cookies that contain not only refined flour but refined sugar and plenty of fat as well. Unrefined grains aren't apt to set off cravings, and they're only high in calories when accompanied by fats (as in fried rice or a muffin made with eggs and butter).

When you eat out, having a refined carbohydrate dish (white pasta or white rice, for example) is a reasonable compromise. You haven't blown anything. This is one way that your eating can alter slightly to fit your life, instead of altering your life to fit your eating.

Don't "overwheat." There are plenty of delicious grains around in addition to wheat, the one we use most in this country. Its protein, gluten, is hard for many people to deal with. Aside from a full-blown gluten allergy or intolerance (the gastric condition *celiac disease* is the most serious of these), a lot of people have some low-level difficulty with wheat. Either they don't feel that they digest it well, or it seems to create excess mucus (dairy is worse on this score, but wheat can be a problem for some people), or they feel tired every day after having a sandwich for lunch. If this is the case with you, eating whole-wheat products won't help your symptoms. Try going wheat-free and see how you feel.

The Love-Powered Bean Stalk

Like whole grains, legumes are substantial foods. It's not difficult to think of lentil soup or baked beans or chili as a main course. Beans do carry the stigma of being poor folks' food, but they're delicious just the same. And what's wrong with a bargain?

Unfortunately, beans also have to live down their reputation for causing intestinal gas. It's true that they can be a culprit in this way, but there are things you can try to mitigate this: using the quick-soak method (see "Bean Cuisine" later in this chapter); eating beans in simple combinations (for instance, in a meal with only a salad and a non-starchy vegetable); spicing them with the herb savory; and sticking to sprouted beans (see "Sprout Farming" page 157) because sprouts have a different molecular structure than dry beans, making flatulence a non-issue. Simply eating slowly can help as well. There's also a commercial product called Beano (over the counter at pharmacies and health food stores) which, taken before a meal, prevents the problem.

Versatile soy products such as edamame, tofu, soymilk, yogurt, "mock meats," and meaty tempeh tend to be easier to digest than whole, cooked beans. They also enable a newcomer to plant-based eating to make this change for the better without feeling the loss of many familiar foods.

If there are some dishes you really think you'll miss when you eliminate animal products from your diet, write them down. Chances are, there's a reasonable facsimile (probably a soy product) sold commercially or one you can make yourself. I can't read your "miss list" but I can let you know that there are hot dogs, hamburgers, cheeses, milk-like drinks, and even ice creams made from soy (and, to a lesser extent, rice, wheat, and other plants). And many vegetarian cookbooks have recipes for everything from kebabs and chicken salad to sauerbraten and gefilte tofu.

Other legumes can find a place on your menus, too. (For more on cooking with legumes, see "Bean Cuisine" page 166.) For now, write on your sheet three bean dishes you like—even if you've never had them without meat. With plenty of herbs and spices, your pork and beans can be just as good without the pork. Split-pea soup is a tasty winter warmer that doesn't need ham, and great chili is a matter of beans, sauce, and seasonings, not ground beef. Just write down your favorite bean dishes to remind yourself that you'd probably like to have them more often. (If you're curious about my list, it's Boston baked beans, taco salad with chili beans, and my mom's black beans and rice—all meatless and all really good.)

Remember the following facts about legumes:

- Dried beans and peas are solid and filling. They will help ease your transition from heavy foods and excess foods to lighter eating overall.
- Soybeans and most of the products made from them are higher in fat than other legumes. Look for fat-reduced tofu (a third less fat) and aseptic packs of one percent low-fat tofu.
- Legumes are a concentrated protein source. For this reason, don't overdo it. A cup of legumes a day is about right.
- If you haven't cooked beans much before, you may want to look into prepackaged bean soups and rice and bean combinations that come with their own seasoning packets.
- It's OK to use canned beans, but if you need to keep your sodium intake especially low, you'll want to drain and rinse them, or buy canned beans at a natural food store where they come with little or no added salt.
- Many bean dishes at non-vegetarian restaurants have some kind of pork in them, and a few Mexican restaurants still use lard in their refried beans. Ask before you order.

Putting It Together

When your fridge and pantry are filled with vegetables, fruits, whole grains, and legumes, you'll be ready for delicious meals that will nourish your body and free your mind to pursue all the inedible—and, in fact, incredible—joys of life. Meal planning will not be a major issue.

I like to have a basic food plan that provides me with some structure (though not too rigid) so I don't have to think much about food. Now that I'm eating more raw food, I start the day with freshly made green juice and have fresh fruit later in the morning. Lunch is a big—trust me on this one: really big—salad with a couple of flax crackers, and dinner is another large salad with a raw soup or a vegetable/nut-based raw entrée, or a simple cooked dish such as a baked potato and/or steamed broccoli. For years leading up to this, though, my breakfast in summer was a fruit smoothie or shake, and in the colder seasons hot cereal with dried fruit, cold cereal with soy or almond milk, a bran muffin, or toast with fruit preserves. On Sundays or holidays, I'd often make pancakes or eggless French toast.

Both in the recent past and now, I make a big salad right after breakfast so it's ready for lunch. I put in chickpeas or avocado and raisins so there's more to the salad than simply greens, and I eat it with flax crackers. Other simple lunches you might consider are leftovers from the previous night's dinner, a sandwich (a mixture of raw and sautéed vegetables in a tortilla is quick and delicious), or hot soup. If you make a big pot of soup on the weekend, you have it available throughout the week. Every now and then instant soup is OK, too—there are some tasty ones at health food stores—with whole-grain rolls, raw vegetables, and bean or tofu dip. These foods travel well, too. You can put soup in a Thermos, salad in a plastic storage container, and sandwiches in waxed paper with the tomato packed separately to avoid soggy bread.

Dinner can be a large salad; an entrée based on whole grains, legumes, or potatoes; and a steamed vegetable. If you want dessert—apple crisp or nondairy ice cream—enjoy, just not too often.

You may be saying, "Rolls? Potatoes? Apple crisp? That's OK for you: You're not trying to lose weight. But what about me?" Let me assure you that this is precisely how I did lose weight. It was never dieting, though, because with the generous assistance of unconditional love, my eating went from inappropriate to appropriate. I ate the food needed by a person with a normal-sized body and my body became normal-sized. I eat the same way today and I remain a normal size. Although you're likely to release weight quite easily after you begin to eat this way, it's not a quick-weight-loss scheme. It's a way of life that's meant to be for life.

Out to Eat

There's no question that eating at home is the surest way to know that the food you're eating is what you think it is. (I'm thinking of the strawberry-banana smoothie I ordered a while back that contained neither strawberries nor bananas but rather some synthetic "smoothie mix.") Still, most people enjoy eating out and you can certainly enjoy it on a love-powered diet.

Ethnic restaurants are the most fun because the cuisines of Italy, China, Thailand, India, Ethiopia, and the Middle East feature numerous dishes that are totally vegetarian. Moreover, you can eat well at almost any restaurant. Most have at least one vegetarian dish on the menu. Salad bars are healthy if you just avoid anything laden with mayonnaise or oil. Steak houses always have baked potatoes and some kind of salad and side vegetables, as do most diners. Meatless burgers have found their way to most mid-scale restaurants' menus. Mexican places can do bean burritos and veggie fajitas without cheese, and even Burger King offers a veggie burger (so does McDonald's, but only in select markets).

At elite restaurants, the chef and other personnel will usually go out of their way to provide you with a vegetable plate or special pasta dish or salad, even in those rare cases when there isn't one on the menu. Wherever you're eating, graciously ask for what you need and expect to get it. If you're flying internationally (or in first class where you can still expect the luxury of food) you can reserve a pure vegetarian meal when you make your reservations. (Reconfirm this twenty-four hours before your flight.) You can also make an advance request for a vegetarian meal for almost any banquet or catered dinner.

I've had very acceptable meals in some very diverse situations. Once I attended a posh dinner reception after a movie premier to write about the event for a magazine. I'd phoned the country club ahead of time to ask for vegetarian food. When the vegetable plate arrived, looking like the cover of a fine cookery magazine, my black-tied tablemates were obviously disappointed with their filet mignon. Several asked the waiter if there were any extra vegetable plates so they could make a trade.

In a completely different sociological environment, I was hungry in the midst of a trip via Greyhound bus. My dinnertime layover was at a little depot and the only food available was provided by a hot dog vendor outside. He made me a hoagie sandwich of sorts: mustard, ketchup, relish, pickles, onions, and shredded lettuce piled on a frankfurter roll. It wasn't the Ritz, but it had a certain charm.

And some years ago on an extended car trip through the rural West, I was getting awfully tired of eating potatoes, toast, and less-than-fresh salads. I wandered into a truck stop in the wilds of Montana and right there on the menu in bold print was "Avocado and Sprout Sandwich on Dark Rye Bread." Given the setting, this was a surrealistic sandwich, albeit much appreciated.

Whether you're eating in love-powered fashion or not, you'll have some enjoyable experiences in restaurants and some that aren't so great. A bonus of this way of life is that it won't matter very much. You'll find that as your attitude becomes more and more empowered by love, food may be more delicious than ever, but it will definitely be less important.

Among Friends

When you eat with other people, those people and the conversation you share will be the highlights of the occasion, regardless of what is served. Food prepared for guests needs to be simple and inviting. By and large, people enjoy simple food. Even those who have no desire to revamp their own style of eating appreciate a natural, vegetarian meal as a change of pace. I think it also makes them feel that they've done something nice for their bodies, which indeed they have.

When you're invited to be a guest for a meal in someone else's home, know that you've been invited because you're liked, not because you'll clean your plate. Let your friend know that your dietary needs are different now, but make it clear that you don't require special treatment. Salads, breads, and grain and vegetable side dishes are usually more than ample at formal dinners. If the affair is informal, like a buffet or a potluck, select what you want and leave what you don't. Bringing a dish to share is not always appropriate, but most of the time it's a welcome gesture.

People are usually understanding about others' dietary preferences. Give your friends and relatives the opportunity to be understanding of yours. When you adopt a love-powered diet because you love yourself and every living thing, maintaining it is simply not difficult. It's a matter of commitment. You know the quotation, "When one truly commits oneself, Providence moves, too." The commitment has to come first; then doors open that you never knew were there.

Your commitment is not to stick to a diet no matter what. It's rather to be motivated by love—no matter what. You'll see the importance of this in your dealings with those closest to you. If you live with other people, you won't be alone when you alter the way you eat. Ideally, your family members would read this book and come to realize why you're making the changes you are. Perhaps they will want to make some changes themselves.

Or they may see this as one more diet, one more phase. They might be threatened by changes they see in you, even those that they've asked you to make, such as losing weight. Your new way of eating could seem extreme to them, and they may let you know that they think you've gone too far. If this is the case, you can:

- Get the support you need elsewhere
- Eat the way you truly believe is best for you
- Remember to be grateful daily for the people you love, even when they aren't as supportive as you would like
- Refrain from the urge to try to convert anybody

In talking about the inner transformation you're undergoing, your life will speak for you. This is true of your new way of eating as well. Whether it's your trimmer body, your higher energy level, or your improved state of mind, benefits will start to show. People will want what you have.

In the meantime, accept the people around you and be willing to put up with some inconvenience. If another family member usually does the cooking, share your needs with that person and make it clear that you don't want to make extra work for him or her. Be willing to cook some of your own food. Offer to take over kitchen duties a couple of nights a week: This way the regular cook gets a break, and you get to introduce this new way of eating to your family without pushing it.

If you wear the chef's hat most of the time and your family expects meat at dinner, you have to make your own decision as to how to proceed. For the last several years of her life, I cared for the elderly woman who had helped raise me. She didn't eat much meat but at times she got a hankering for bacon or sardines or stewed chicken. Although I was committed to love-powered eating for myself, I fixed those things for her when she asked for them. Shortly before she passed away at age eighty-seven, she told me she realized that being vegetarian was important to me, that preparing her meat had probably been hard, and how much she'd appreciated it.

Some people could say that I'd have shown her—not to mention the animals—more love by giving her healthy vegetarian food without exception. Maybe they're right and in a similar circumstance today, that might be exactly what I'd do. But at the time I was following my heart. What she told me just before she died had a lot more to do with that intangible aspect of the human heart than with bacon or sardines.

When you're healthy and happy and free from obsession, you're also freer to love your family, your friends, and yourself. If you're not yet healthy, happy, and obsession-free, love your family and friends and yourself anyway. That will help you get there.

Love the foods that nourish your body and the life that this nourishment provides you. Love your fullness and your emptiness. Most of all, love God, by whatever name you choose, and see your emptiness filled and your fullness redeemed. When you love like this, you'll soon discover that you're no longer eating to fill a bottomless pit, solve a hopeless problem, or squelch a nameless fear. You'll be eating to live.

Culinary Basics

Your personal cooking style can be part of your solution just as it may have been part of your problem. Food addicts who are good cooks often allow their disease to take over that talent. They spend most of their time in the kitchen and specialize in preparing their binge foods. In recovery, however, people with a gift for food preparation can use it to put together beautiful works of art, creating healthful meals for themselves and for those they love. Since they're cooking because they want to and not because an obsession is forcing them to do it, the kitchen becomes one of many places for them to express creativity, artistry, and love.

On the other hand, there are food addicts who detest cooking. They stock up for binges at convenience stores and fast-food eateries, and in a pinch they can binge on anything in the kitchen that requires no preparation. When these people get well, they're not apt to become gourmet chefs. They can turn their lack of interest in cooking to an advantage, emphasizing simplicity in their meals.

To Market, to Market

You can put love in your diet and be well-nourished if you shop only at your local supermarket. Hit the produce department first; you'll do most of your shopping there. Then make brief stops at frozen foods and other strategic points within the store. There will be entire sections you'll bypass, like the butcher counter and the aisles of snack foods and soda. Grocery shopping will get much quicker and easier. You'll probably notice that your food bill will decrease as well.

You may want to make quick stops at the store for small amounts of food rather than make huge hauls every couple of weeks. After coming in a from a trip last year, I remember stopping at the market for mesclun greens, fresh vegetable soup prepared by the deli staff, a lovely round loaf of whole-grain bread, organic raspberries (on sale!), a bottle of sparkling cider, and a bouquet of mixed flowers. It made the perfect welcome-home supper, with bread and soup left over for the next day's lunch and enough floral cheerfulness to last a week. I find that whirlwind shopping trips like this are more pleasant than stocking up for the apocalypse.

Find out what days the store gets its produce deliveries and make those your shopping days. If you prefer to shop only once a week, use the more delicate produce like spring greens and asparagus first and the heartier vegetables like kale and carrots later.

Although it's not mandatory, getting acquainted with the stock of a good natural foods store will make your meals more interesting. This is where you're most likely to find vegetarian specialty items: egg substitute to be used in baking, a wide variety of meatless burgers, the kind of soymilk you like, and types of grains and beans that aren't available at many grocery stores. You can also expect to find more organically grown grains, beans, and produce than at a store catering to a general clientele.

Some of the prices at health food stores may seem high, but you'll get value for your money and in many cases support small, careful companies whose profit margins are meager for the quality they offer. In some cases, you can actually save money at a health food store, and when you buy grains, flour, and nuts from bulk bins, you can choose the exact quantity you want and avoid paying for expensive packaging.

A real money-saver for the energetic is a food co-op. There are storefront co-ops and private buying clubs that you can join. By working for the co-op a few hours a month, you can buy your food at a hefty savings. (Being part of a co-op is also a way to meet other people who are interested in living more naturally and healthfully.)

Supermarkets are getting smarter, and many offer an array of organic produce and bulk products. Get yourself an imaginary shopping cart and we'll make the weekly grocery run. Don't feel that you would have to buy all of this on a real shopping trip; this is for practice. The sample list below includes most of the items called for in common vegetarian recipes, and I've stuck with those foods that are most widely available throughout North America. If there are other vegetables, fruits, whole grains, and legumes that you like, add them to the list. And if there are items listed that you don't like, that don't agree with you, or that are binge foods for you, make a different selection.

Produce

- Apples
- Bananas
- Broccoli and other greens (kale, collards, Swiss chard, spinach)
- Cabbage, red or green
- Carrots
- Celery
- Lettuce (preferably leaf or romaine; iceberg is less nutritious)
- Mushrooms (try specialty mushrooms like oyster, enoki, Chinese wood ear, and shiitake)
- Onions (scallions, too, if you like them)
- Oranges, grapefruit, lemons
- Other seasonal fruits and berries
- Sweet red or yellow bell peppers

- Potatoes, yams, winter squash
- Specialty greens (arugula, cilantro, radicchio) and pre-washed-and-packaged salads
- Tomatoes

Frozen Food

- Frozen lemon juice
- Fruit juice concentrate
- Unsweetened frozen berries (for thick, frosty smoothies)
- Vegetables of your choice (plain, no fancy sauces)

Canned Goods

- Beans (such as pintos, chickpeas, chili beans in sauce, and vegetarian baked beans)
- Soups (optional—most canned soups are quite salty; choose vegetable, lentil, and minestrone soups without chicken or beef broth)
- Tomatoes
- Tomato sauce and paste

Packaged Foods

- All-fruit jam or preserves (no added sugar)
- Aluminum-free baking powder (Rumford's is one brand)
- Apple cider vinegar or seasoned rice vinegar (the latter stands on its own as a delicate fat-free, calorie-free salad dressing), mustard, natural soy sauce (look for reduced-sodium tamari)
- Brown rice (get the regular and quick-cooking kind), rice pilaf, and flavorful white rice like jasmine and basmati (whole grains are generally preferred but white rice works better in certain dishes and is easier than brown rice for some people to digest)
- Dried beans and peas (lentils, split peas, navy beans, or your choice)

- Dry cereal (look for whole grains and a low sugar content; avoid granola unless it's specified low-fat)
- Herbs and spices of your choice (Mrs. Dash is a good salt-free seasoning; the most popular spices used in vegetarian cooking are garlic, ground black pepper, onion powder, basil, oregano, cumin, chili powder, curry, parsley flakes, and paprika—sweet Hungarian paprika is best)
- Natural peanut butter, English walnuts, and slivered almonds
- Nutritional yeast flakes (a high-B-complex supplement powder included in some vegan recipes for its cheesy taste)
- Oatmeal (quick or old-fashioned)
- Olive oil (look for cold-pressed oil; use the extra virgin oil in salad dressings, and use all oils sparingly)
- Pasta (use some that's wholegrain)
- Raisins or other dried fruit, if desired (without the sulfur dioxide, which is sometimes used as a preservative)
- Real maple syrup and/or agave nectar
- Rice cakes, whole-grain crackers, and popcorn to pop in your air-popper
- Seltzer
- Teas (black and herbal), coffee and/or Postum or Teeccino (grain coffee substitutes)
- Vegetable broth (this comes in aseptic boxes)
- Whole-wheat bread (read the label: "wheat flour," "flour," and "enriched flour" all mean white; look for one hundred percent whole wheat)
- Whole-wheat flour (if you bake yeast bread, using part unbleached white flour may be a good transitional step)
- Whole-wheat pastry flour (for quick breads and muffins)

Refrigerated Foods

- Tofu (a refrigerated food but likely to be found in the produce section; also look for one percent low-fat tofu—Mori-Nu is a common brand name—in aseptic packaging)
- Whole-wheat and/or corn tortillas (sometimes frozen)

- Yeast, if you bake (note that baking yeast and nutritional or brewer's yeast are entirely different and not interchangeable)

Natural Food Glossary

The fruits and vegetables with which you're already familiar are true natural foods, and a healthful diet doesn't demand a boundless repertoire of different grains and legumes.

Nevertheless, becoming acquainted with some of the more unusual foods can give your meals welcome variety. Some of these, tofu for example, can also be used to create dishes reminiscent of those you no longer eat and may miss. You don't have to eat any of these things, but they're available at health food stores and some supermarkets for you to try:

Agar. A vegetarian gelatin made from seaweed. Agar, also called agar-agar, comes in sticks or flakes (the flakes yield the most consistent results). Use it like ordinary gelatin; one tablespoon of flakes will gel one cup of liquid.

Agave nectar. A sweet, golden syrup from a cactus plant. It's used like honey but, unlike most nutritive sweeteners, agave is low on the Glycemic Index.

Almond milk. This light, delicious beverage can be used anywhere milk is called for. It's lower in calories than skim, soy, or rice milk. Brands include Pacific (organic) and Blue Diamond.

Buckwheat. A hearty, quick-cooking grain with an earthy flavor. Also known as kasha, buckwheat can be cooked whole as a breakfast cereal or as a substitute for rice. As a flour, it's most popular in pancakes.

Egg substitute. Powder to stand in for eggs in baking. Use one teaspoon of egg substitute whisked with two tablespoons of water for each egg. (Ener-G and Jolly Joan are two brand names.)

Granular sweeteners. Date sugar is ground, dehydrated dates. It has a full-flavored taste, something like dark brown sugar. Sucanat is made from sugar-cane juice that has been dehydrated and milled into a powder. It's richly flavored and very good in quick breads and bran muffins. Stevia is a calorie-free herbal sweetener available in both granular and liquid forms.

Millet. Little rounded golden grains that cook up light and fluffy. Use as you would use rice at dinnertime, as a hot breakfast cereal, or as a base for other dishes such as vegetarian loaves and burgers. (And throw millet instead of rice at newlyweds, since it won't harm the birds that eat it.)

Miso. Salty, fermented paste made from cooked, aged soybeans and sometimes from grains. Thick and spreadable, it's used for flavoring a wide variety of dishes and for making soup bases. Mellow white miso has the mildest flavor and makes the ideal introduction.

Nut butters. Spreads made from almonds, walnuts, cashews, sunflower seeds, pumpkin seeds, and peanuts. These are high in fat, but they can be used in moderation and in the preparation of other dishes. One that you'll see called for in recipes fairly often is tahini, made from sesame seeds.

Nutritional yeast. Imparts a sharp, cheesy flavor to sauces, soups, and casseroles. It can also be sprinkled on toast, popcorn, or spaghetti. Yeast flakes taste much better than the powder. Either form is rich in B-complex vitamins and many brands are fortified with vitamin B12.

Quinoa. Round, sand-colored grain with a mild, nutty taste and fascinating history going back to the ancient Incan culture. It cooks quickly and contains all essential amino acids.

Ramen noodles. Dry, wavy noodles that need only to be boiled or steamed for a few minutes to reconstitute their texture and be ready to eat. They come in packages with seasoning included for a nearly instant meal. Conventional varieties are high in fat, full of chemical additives and made from refined grains. Get yours *only* at the health food store.

Raw cashews. Nuts, or more technically the fruit of the cashew tree, raw cashews are white and quite unlike roasted, salted cashews. High in fat, these are "rich relatives" like all nuts, but they're extremely versatile and relatively small amounts of them can be used to make "milk," white sauce, gravy, and a variety of other dishes. Buy the pieces rather than whole cashews to save money.

Rice milk. Milk-like beverage made from rice. It's light and slightly sweet. Fortified rice milk is available with added calcium. (The brand name is Rice Dream.)

Seitan. Chewy, high-protein food made from baked or boiled wheat gluten. Seitan tastes much like meat when used in stews and casseroles or barbecued on a bun.

Soymilk. This milk-like beverage made from soybeans is hardly an "alternative" any more, now that soymilk is available in grocery stores and coffee bars. Buy organic soymilk (and all soy products) to be sure you're not ingesting a genetically modified product. The fat content varies; look for the light varieties. Enriched soymilk contains added calcium, B12, and other nutrients.

Tamari. Natural soy sauce, fragrant, flavorful, and far superior to typical grocery store soy sauce. Traditional tamari is wheat-free. Soy sauce made from soy and wheat is called shoyu. Nama shoyu is unheated and suitable for raw-fooders. These seasonings are very salty, but reduced-sodium tamari is less so.

Tempeh. A fermented soy product of Indonesian heritage. Tempeh is very meaty in texture, barbecues beautifully, and is a natural for chili. Like most soy foods, it's fairly high in fat.

Tofu. Soybean curd that has made its way from Chinese restaurant menus to most supermarkets. This white cake is virtually flavorless on its own so it takes on the character of the condiments used with it. It can serve as the "meat" in a stir-fry, the "sour cream" in stroganoff, or the "cream cheese" in cheesecake. Look for reduced-fat versions. (See "Tofu 101" later in this chapter.)

Wheat-free breads and pastas. Breads, noodles, and spaghetti made from rice, quinoa, corn, and other grains. Wheat is a common allergen and many people are sensitive to wheat gluten. Health food stores stock breads, crackers, and pastas that contain no wheat.

Going Organic

One way to show some extra love to yourself, the children of the world, wildlife, and the Earth itself is to purchase at least some of your food organically grown. If you have some resistance to this idea, you're not alone: I held out for a long time. It seemed to me that only health fanatics, leftover hippies, and the people my grandmother used to say had "more money than sense" would pay the usually high price for organic groceries. I figured that I was doing all right with regular food.

That was before I realized that synthetic insecticides, herbicides, and fertilizers weren't "regular" until some sixty years ago. Chemical-treated agriculture is a relatively recent phenomenon that came on the scene after World War II. (The pesticide *methyl parathion*, for example, was developed by the Nazis as a lethal nerve gas. Sixty times more toxic than DDT, its use is banned or restricted in twenty-three countries, including the U.S. as of 1999, but it's still applied elsewhere to grains, produce, and cotton.)

And although the use of insecticides in agriculture has increased twelve times over the past forty years, damage to crops from pests has doubled during this time. Research from France now suggests that some ammonia fertilizers and certain pesticides may prevent plants from absorbing micronutrients. "This not only makes them less nutritious," says agricultural economist Terry Gips, author of *Breaking the Pesticide Habit*, "but it weakens the plant much like an immune deficiency, so insects can come to affect the weaker plants. It's a catch-22: the more you use, the more you have to use."

But consumers can opt for the organic alternative. Gips offers the follow reasons for making the switch:

- *Personal health.* Conventionally grown food contains residues of various pesticides. A Natural Resources Defense Council study found that forty-four percent of California's fresh produce contained residues of nineteen of these, including proven carcinogens.
- *Social justice.* Nursing mothers in Central America have DDT in their breast milk at levels forty-two times the World Health Organization's standards as a result of aerial spraying and residues in foods. In the United States, the National Cancer Institute found that farmers in Nebraska and Kansas who were exposed to the herbicide 2, 4-D ran six times the risk of developing non-Hodgkins lymphoma.
- *Wildlife protection.* Runoff from agricultural chemicals concentrates in ponds, contaminating the food and water of migrating waterfowl and resulting in deformities.
- *Ecology.* Growing crops organically doesn't contaminate the ground or surface water, and it saves energy since synthetic pesticides and fertilizers are made

from petrochemicals (petroleum). Synthetic fertilizers also cause nitrates, which break down into carcinogenic nitrosamines, to enter groundwater. (A U.S. Environmental Protection Agency study showed that more than fifty percent of wells tested contain nitrates.) Organic methods also cause far less soil erosion, and organic farmers rotate their crops, which produces richer soil. Natural nitrogen fertilizers also make soil stronger, unlike artificial nitrogen, which breaks down humus, making it susceptible to loss from wind and rain. "Up to five bushels of topsoil can be lost for each bushel of corn conventionally grown," says Gips.

- *Economics.* Economies of scale in transportation and marketing means that the more people buy organic foods, the less those foods will cost. And demand encourages supply. Every additional customer helps create the demand that will encourage more growers to farm organically. Health food stores carry organically grown grains, nuts, legumes, and often fresh fruits and vegetables. Food co-ops make these available at a lower cost. Organic produce and some other foods are available at quite a few supermarkets, as well; even the giant Wal-Mart has joined this party.

Look for foods labeled "certified organic." The word *natural* has no legal definition. It's usually applied to products with no synthetic colorings, flavorings, preservatives, or other artificial additives. That's good, but it says nothing about the way in which the food was grown. *Certified organic* means that an independent monitoring agency has inspected a farm and determined that no synthetic fertilizers or pesticides have been used there in the past three years and that the farmer practices good soil management.

Now, I can't tell you that you'll lose more weight or eat less obsessively when you fill your market basket organically. I do happen to believe that organically grown foods taste better. Maybe that's just because I like the way I feel about myself when I eat them. Or maybe some of the special care and attention that the farmers give the soil comes through in the rice and the carrots and the apples.

I also find that choosing organic foods puts me in closer touch with nature, with the land, and with my part in all that's natural. Feeling connected in this way brings with it a balance that's antithetical to obsessing over anything. If paying an extra forty cents a pound for tomatoes can give me that, I'm getting quite a bargain.

The Art of the Salad

A salad doesn't have to be token greenery, bland and perfunctory. In fact, it doesn't even have to be what we think of as salad. You can serve light and nutritious raw vegetables as:

- *Crudités.* Carrots, celery, peppers, zucchini, broccoli, cauliflower, jicama (a starchy root), cucumbers, kohlrabi, mushrooms, and thinly sliced turnips are great alone or with dip. (With a beginner's book on garnishing and a few simple tools, you can make edible artworks from raw veggies.)
- *Sandwich fillers.* Salad sandwiches are standard fare in Britain, especially ones made with cucumbers or watercress. Make a jolly good veggie sandwich yourself by stuffing some vegetables into a pita, rolling them in a tortilla, or skipping the starch in favor of a wrap using a romaine leaf as the wrapper.
- *One-dish meals.* Make them a main course by adding cooked beans (try garbanzos or spiced chili beans), brown rice, steamed new potatoes, curly pasta or elbow macaroni, or tofu cubes (marinate them in three parts water to two parts natural tamari soy sauce). Include bread or rolls on the side if you wish.

There's an art to the traditional tossed salad as well. You can experiment on your own or use recipes, but here are general guidelines for a salad you'll actually want to eat:

Choose vegetables that are in season. Or pick imported produce that looks fresh and appetizing. Go with colors, textures, and flavors that complement each other. Visualize a salad made from iceberg lettuce, peeled cucumber, cauliflower, and mushrooms. There's no color there, no appeal. Now picture a salad with bright red tomato wedges, a cucumber crinkle-cut with its green edge intact, cauliflower set off by grated carrots and a few ripe olives, and mushrooms tossed with spinach as green as a St. Patrick's Day hat. Now that's better.

Wash the vegetables you've chosen. Pay close attention to leafy ones like spinach and arugula that collect sediment in their crevices. Dry them before putting them in your salad bowl. If you use a wooden salad bowl, rub its interior with a cut garlic clove. This will impart a wonderful flavor to your salad.

Go easy on the oil. The main purpose of using oil in salad is to help herbs and seasonings cling to the vegetables. A tablespoon in a very large salad is sufficient for that. Try spraying on oil from a pump bottle instead pouring it on.

You can actually do without oil altogether if you toss your greens with lemon or lime juice. Sprinkle amply with salt-free seasonings and seasoned salt like Spike (if desired). Seasoned rice vinegar is a superb dressing on its own. Using cut tomato slices also provides liquid for this no-dressing dressing.

Avocado is another useful addition. Although high in oil content, it comes packed with the vitamins, minerals, and fiber of a *whole* food—something even the best bottled oil can't claim. Avocado also makes a salad more filling than any dressing.

You can also dress up a salad with tasty garnishes such as steamed vegetables (asparagus, string beans, broccoli) and small quantities of tasty "rich relatives" like sunflower seeds and olives. Or try topping a salad with whatever else is on the menu, like vegetarian chili or baked beans.

Make it easy to eat salad. Keep washed vegetables in your refrigerator at all times. Salad tastes best when you eat it right after you put it together, but if you need to, make your lunch salad after breakfast and keep it in an airtight bowl until noontime. (If using dressing, add it right before you eat.)

Treat yourself to fresh fruit salads. Keep them simple: a melon salad of cubed cantaloupe, honeydew, and casaba melon; a tropical salad of pineapple, tangerine slices, and bananas; or an autumn salad of apples, grapes, and pears. If you use apples or bananas, add a squeeze of lemon to keep their colors true. Make a meal of a fruit salad with the addition of a cashew cream (eighth of a cup of raw cashew pieces to four ounces of fresh orange juice, blended until smooth) and a sprinkling of sunflower seeds, raisins, or chopped dates.

Sprout Farming

You don't need a back forty or even a backyard to grow organic produce of your own. That's because sprout farming can be done anywhere. Even if you skip the alfalfa sprouts on salad bars and can take or leave the mung bean sprouts in Chinese food, you're apt to become much fonder of these "baby vegetables" if you grow them yourself.

Sprouts are seeds that have just begun to germinate, and these tiny plants are bursting with enzymes, vitamins, and minerals while shy on calories. Start with good organic seeds (get edible seeds and beans from a health food store, not chemically treated seeds meant for gardening) and count on a hefty return—at least 5 pounds—of sprouts from every pound of seeds. Among the sprouts you can easily grow are:

- *Alfalfa.* Use raw in salads. These sprout in two to five days.
- *Dried whole peas.* Surprisingly sweet and crunchy, these need two to three days to grow to be ready for salads, snacking, or steaming.
- *Lentils.* They take two to three days to sprout and are good raw or cooked; use them in soups and stir-fries.
- *Peanuts.* My all-time favorite, peanut sprouts, are low in fat since the sprouting process requires energy and gets it from the oil present in the unsprouted seed. These sprouts are ready in two days, no more than three. (Only raw peanuts will sprout.)
- *Radishes.* Spicy. These will perk up an uneventful salad any day. Give them three to five days' growing time.
- *Sunflower seeds.* These sprout almost as deliciously as peanuts. They are leafy and crunchy at the same time and excellent in salads or on sandwiches.

You can also grow mung bean sprouts in two to four days, but since removing the bitter hulls is tedious, you may prefer to purchase these already sprouted and hulled in the produce section of your supermarket or at an Asian grocery.

Wheat and other whole grains sprout, too. They can be cooked when barely germinated (after the night's soaking and one day's sprouting time) or used raw as a strangely sweet sprout when allowed to grow for four to five days.

Soybeans are nearly impossible to sprout at home, but the soy sprouts that you can buy at Asian markets are tasty and substantial. These cannot be eaten raw; stir-fry them.

To grow a sprout garden, all you'll need are a Mason jar (a used peanut butter jar will do, unless you want a lot of sprouts; then use something the size of the large institutional food jars you can get from a restaurant or school), a piece of cheese-cloth, and a rubber band. Then follow these steps:

1. Soak the seeds (one type at a time unless sprouting times are similar) in the jar overnight, or for at least six hours. It's important to use distilled or spring water for this purpose since chlorinated water can impair sprouting.
2. Cover with a piece of cheesecloth and attach with a rubber band. Drain the seeds and rinse them with fresh water (tap water is fine for this). You'll want the seeds damp, not wet.
3. Turn the jar on its side at the edge of a sink or in a dish drainer. Rinse and drain twice a day until you're ready to harvest. (It's also a good idea to grow your sprouts in the dark—in a cupboard or beneath a dishtowel—until the last day, when you'll place them in a sunny window to develop chlorophyll and nice green leaves.)

As you may imagine, children love to grow sprouts. And when they grow them, they'll want to eat them.

A Steamy Romance with Vegetables

Lightly steamed vegetables taste delicious and take no talent on the cook's part. Steaming is also the most nutrient-saving cooking method. Your cookware set probably comes with a double-boiler that can be used for steaming, Otherwise, pick up a stainless-steel steaming trivet available in any cookware department for just a couple of dollars (or at the 99-cent store for half that). Simply place washed vegetables, whole or cut, in the basket over boiling water. The water shouldn't touch the vegetables. Cover tightly and steam until they're bright and tender-crisp. When preparing vegetables that require longer cooking, check the water level and add more water if it boils away. Here are steaming times for some popular vegetables.

Vegetable Steaming Times

Vegetable	*Steaming Time (min.)*
Beets (medium, whole)	30–40
Beets (sliced)	5–6
Broccoli	10–15
Brussels sprouts	10–15
Butternut squash	20–30
Cabbage	10–20
Carrots (sliced)	10–15
Carrots (whole)	20–30
Collard greens	8–12
Green peas, pea pods	5–10
Kale	5–10
String beans	12–15
Sweet potatoes (small to medium, whole)	25–30
White potatoes (small to medium, whole)	25–30
Zucchini	1–15

Stir-frying is another cooking method that's quick, easy, and produces a nutritious result. Unlike deep-frying, this technique doesn't require a large amount of oil. Less than a tablespoon should be enough in a heavy skillet, no-stick pan, or wok. Spread the oil over the surface of the pan and cook quickly, adding other liquids—water, sherry (or apple juice), tomato juice, or sodium-reduced tamari—and stir constantly. If you add extra water and cover intermittently, you're steam-frying, which is a good way to get maximum flavor with minimum fat.

Soup Stock

An organization that wanted a vegetarian luncheon for a seminar was told by a hotel chef, "You cannot make soup without chicken broth." They changed hotels and got terrific soup—without the chicken broth. You can make terrific soup, too. Your stock options include readymade vegetable broth (in the soup aisle at the grocery store); a broth you make yourself from hot water and miso (the fermented soy product we talked about earlier); or from hot water and a powdered vegetable broth mix or bouillon (brands include Vogue and Seitenbacher). Some of the powdered stocks taste like chicken or beef, if you're looking for that familiar flavor.

If you want to take the homemade route, you can make a stock as good as your grandmother's by following this recipe: Save vegetable scraps and the water left from steaming vegetables. With the exception of cabbage-family members, such as broccoli and cauliflower, any vegetables will do. Scrubbed potato peelings are really good, and so are the ends of beans and the tips of carrots.

You can use onions, garlic, and mushrooms, too. Add your scraps (and any other vegetables you're using) to boiling water—about two cups of vegetables to four cups of water—and up to half a teaspoon of salt. Cover the pot and let the stock simmer just below the boiling point for about an hour. Let it cool; then strain and discard the vegetables.

Your stock will last in the refrigerator for one week, or you can freeze it in ice-cube trays. Use it as a base for all kinds of soups: corn chowder, garden vegetable, lentil, minestrone, navy bean, split pea, or potato. You can make cream soups by using unsweetened non-dairy milk (almond, oat, or soy), tahini (sesame butter), or blended raw cashews to impart a creamy texture. You can also blend portions of a non-cream soup such as fresh pea or vegetable, add a thickener like arrowroot or cornstarch, and reheat—stirring until it reaches the consistency you're looking for.

Soups are one of the best reasons for having winter; and cold soups, like gazpacho and fruit soups, are delightful when it's hot.

Veggie by Brand—Some Prepared Foods to Try

. . . .

While fresh foods should comprise the bulk of your diet, we all need some convenience sometimes, and these items—a mere introduction to all that's out there—can fit the bill. This list also includes helpful transition foods to cover the place on the plate where the animal products used to be. While all these products are vegetarian, not every item in these brands' lines is strictly vegan; read the labels.

Except when otherwise noted, you can purchase these items at Whole Foods, Trader Joe's, Ralph's, Kroger, Albertson's, and other national chains, as well as your local health food store. You may also want to check out the site www.match-meats.com, a company that makes extremely authentic vegan versions of ground pork, beef, and chicken, Italian sausage, and breakfast sausage—even—crabmeat.

Refrigerated Section

Earth Balance—nondairy "butter"—no trans fat

Eat in the Raw—Parma! Parmesan cheese alternative

Follow Your Heart—Vegan Gourmet Cheese Alternative (the only vegan cheese I know of that melts; the mozzarella can go on pizza)

Gimme Lean—sausage

Lightlife—anything they make, especially their soy Chik'n Strips, Soy Steak Strips, and Smart Bacon. Also, deli meats like soy ham, bologna, salami, turkey, and pepperoni (Old World Bologna is the best)

Silk—soymilk (including a low-fat variety) and non-dairy creamer

Morningstar Farms Meal Starters—Steak Strips and Chik'n Strips

Soy Boy—Courage Burgers. Very reasonably priced. Put in the toaster—good "kid food"

Sunergia Soyfoods—soy feta (any gourmet could put this on a cheese tray)

Tofutti—cream cheese, sour cream, and American cheese slices (watch the fat here)

Turtle Island Foods—Tofurky Deli Slices (the smoked turkey is terrific)

WhiteWave—Baked Tofu, ready to eat and great for sandwiches or to chop and use as the "meat" in a chef's salad

Whole Soy—yogurt and cream cheese style soy spread

Yves—mock meats, most low in fat: Canadian Bacon, Chick'n Nuggets, Smart Dogs (veggie hotdogs)

Zensoy—Pudding in little cups of reasonable portion size

On the Shelf

Amy's—No Chicken Noodle Soup

Veggie by Brand—Some Prepared Foods to Try (*continued*)

. . . .

Cucamonga—Agave Nectar Light (looks and tastes like honey)

Dr. McDougall's Right Foods—Instant soups, light oatmeal, pancake mix

Ener-G—Egg Replacer

Fantastic World Foods—Sloppy Joe Mix; Tofu Scrambler. Fast and cheap!

Follow Your Heart—Vegenaise (mayo)

Ghirardelli's—dark chocolate

Nasoya—Nayonaise (mayo), also vegan salad dressings

Pacific Natural Foods—Almond milk, vegetable broth

Vegan Supreme—marshmallows

Worthington—Tuno Fish

Frozen Section

Amy's—soy cheese pizza, tofu lasagna, non-dairy vegetable pot pie

Boca—Boca Burgers (original vegan), soy chicken and sausage, Boca Burger Crumbles (ground beef replacement)

Follow Your Heart—Chicken Free Chicken

Gardenburger—veggie burgers, Chik'n, and Riblets (fake ribs)

Health Is Wealth—Pizza Munchies and Chicken-free Nuggets

Nate's—Meatless Meatballs

Soy Boy—Tofu ravioli

Soy Delicious—"Decadence" line, gourmet ice cream (a great substitute for the real thing, but if ice cream was a binge inducer, this probably will be, too)

Soy Dream—ice cream, very authentic, caveat as above

Turtle Island Foods—Tofurky, subs for the turkey at holiday time for the whole family or those vegetarians present

The Perfect Potato (and Toppers)

To bake the perfect potato (or a darned good one at least), bypass the microwave. Choose firm russet or yellow Finn potatoes and cut out any "eyes." Prick the skins several times with a fork and bake in a baking dish (this seems to be the secret) in an oven preheated to 450°F. Baking will take about an hour, depending upon the size of the potatoes. If you plan to stuff them with other vegetables, they should be fairly large. You can lightly oil the skins if you "want to," but don't wrap your potatoes in aluminum foil. There's some evidence that cooking in foil and with aluminum cookware can cause aluminum build-up in the body.

The perfect potato deserves the proper topper. Butter is an animal product and, for all intents and purposes, straight, saturated fat. Ditto sour cream. If you use margarine, make sure that it's dairy-free and contains no trans-fatty acids, which behave in the body like cholesterol-elevating saturated fat. Or go with one of the following unorthodox but tasty toppings:

- Salsa—homemade or from a jar
- Broccoli—over-steamed so you can mash it (broccoli stems left after you've cooked the flowerets work just fine) with plenty of ground black pepper
- Cauliflower—just like broccoli
- Mashed sweet potatoes or yams—no kidding; cold leftovers work fine—sort of like cold butter on a hot potato
- Marinara sauce—with plenty of garlic and basil (or a cheese-free pesto)
- Barbecue sauce—those at health food stores have no refined sugar
- Steak sauce—at restaurants, steak sauce or mustard is sometimes the best you can do, but they're really not bad
- Ratatouille—sautéed vegetables with tomato sauce, my favorite tater topper
- Avocados—mashed or thinly sliced or seasoned with lemon juice, cumin, and cayenne for guacamole
- Flax oil—a light luscious oil providing omega-3 fatty acids and yummy on baked or mashed potatoes, corn on the cob, toast or waffles—even popcorn. Purchase plain, pure flaxseed oil, not one fortified with additional nutrients or flavored in any way. Spectrum Essentials makes a simple, organic flaxseed oil. I use it regularly. Flax oil is highly perishable so keep it refrigerated and use prior to its expiration date.

Combine these with other seasonings, like lemon-pepper, Italian herbs, powdered vegetable broth, sweet Hungarian paprika, scallions, or chives, and find your own specialties. A potato is fairly dry and mild-tasting, so you're looking for something to provide a little moisture and a touch of spice. Use your imagination.

Sandwich Ideas

Every once in while you'll see on a menu the archaic diet plate of cottage cheese, a canned peach half, and a burger without a bun. Not that I'm promoting white flour, but it would be better to have a bun without a burger. A decent sandwich can, however, be well-filled and come with the bun or both pieces of bread. There are, in fact, a variety of breads from which to choose.

- Whole-wheat or whole-rye bread, whole-spelt bread, or a gluten-free specialty bread if you're sensitive to wheat
- Whole-grain pita pocket
- Whole-wheat English muffin
- Whole-wheat burger bun
- Whole-wheat bagel
- Whole-wheat kaiser roll
- Whole-wheat or corn tortillas
- Other unleavened breads—matzo, Indian chapati, or Ethiopian injera (a flat, spongy bread used as an edible utensil)
- Large crackers—rice cakes, Scottish oatcakes, or Norwegian rye crisp-bread (sold in large rounds)
- A breadless sandwich wrapper such as a romaine or collard leaf

Once you've found the bread (or bread stand-in), you need to fill, top, or spread it. There are dozens of ways to do this, keeping in mind to not overdo the quantities of high-fat or very sweet sandwich fillers. Here are some ideas to get you started.

Hummus. The classic Middle Eastern spread (or dip) of puréed chickpeas and tahini. To keep fat content low, use more chickpeas and less tahini. If you use canned beans, drain off all the water (except what you'll need to get the blender to run) so your spread won't be too thin. Serve hummus or chickpea purée in pita pockets with plenty of crisp, colorful vegetables.

Split-pea spread. Leftover split-pea soup or cooked split peas thicken in the refrigerator overnight for a fine sandwich spread. Add more seasonings if you like. This is especially good on hot toast—it almost melts.

Vegetables. Thinly sliced cucumbers, grated carrots, alfalfa and radish sprouts, lettuce, and sliced tomato are great as stand-alone sandwiches. Try a mix of vegetables on a roll with a thin layer of tofu mayonnaise or Dijon-style mustard, or roll in a tortilla or chapatti (you can use some steamed vegetables, too).

Tempeh. Tempeh makes a meaty sandwich, something like a pork tenderloin but lower in fat. Readymade tempeh burgers and cutlets (some only need to be heated for one minute in a toaster oven) are in the freezer section at health food stores. Tempeh generously doused with barbecue sauce at the end of cooking and rolled in a tortilla burrito-style got rave reviews when a firefighter friend of mine fixed it at the firehouse—hardly what you'd think of as a bastion of vegetarianism.

Fruit spreads. Remember jelly sandwiches from childhood? You can make them again using the fruit-only jams and preserves available at both grocery and health food stores. Or you can mix a dried fruit spread by gently simmering for one hour four cups of chopped dried fruit (prunes, raisins, and dates), one and a half cups of water, a third of a cup of grated carrots, a third of a cup of lemon juice, and half a teaspoon of salt. Purée in your food processor (with a metal "S" blade), and simmer again until it thickens.

Avocado. A quartered, thinly sliced avocado makes a fine sandwich filling when accompanied by hot mustard, tomato slices, and sprouts. Or make guacamole by mashing avocados with chopped tomatoes and onions, garlic, and chili powder; add a squeeze of lemon juice to keep the avocado from turning brown, and salt to taste. Cut the fat content in your guacamole recipe by substituting cold, steamed broccoli for half the avocado.

Burgers. Frozen, meatless burgers are available in both supermarkets and health food stores. My favorite are original-recipe Boca Burgers—fat-free, vegan, and absolutely scrumptious—but there are lots of choices; try them all.

Leftovers. Use the vegetarian loaves and burgers you've made for dinner. Many cookbooks include recipes for these made from grains such as rice or oats with beans or chopped nuts, vegetables, and seasonings. Some can be mashed as is for next-day sandwiches. Others mix well with tofu mayonnaise. (Readymade eggless mayonnaise is also available at health food stores. Check the labels; some are as high in fat as conventional mayonnaise while others are reduced-fat. If you like mustard, you can sometimes use that as a substitute, too.)

Nut butters. Almond butter is my favorite. You can cut the fat content of any nut butter by mixing one tablespoon of it with two tablespoons of water and beating with a fork to emulsify them. You end up with more butter for the same amount of fat. Use nut butter on one slice of bread and fruit spread on the other.

Lettuce and shredded carrots provide a welcome, moist contrast to the dryness of the nut butter and bread. Sliced bananas are really good, too. Serve sandwiches with a lot of raw vegetables, a bowl of soup if you like, and an apple later if you're not quite satisfied. This is an ample and easy lunch—and when you bring it to work, I guarantee no one will ask, "What kind of diet is it this week?"

Bean Cuisine

Whether we don't know beans about something or it doesn't amount to a hill of them, beans are disparaged in metaphor and fact. Actually, this staple food comes in more than fifty varieties and has a 9,000-year history of cultivation that has made it important in nourishing and sustaining the human race.

Legumes are also a top-choice food for the twenty-first century because they're full of fiber and minerals, provide quality protein without the drawbacks of protein from animal sources, and are in most cases very low in fat. They also keep well and are inexpensive. Beans are cheap enough when you buy them, but when you consider that they swell with water during soaking and cooking, you're getting more satiety for the money. That's the opposite of meat, which shrinks when it's cooked, leaving you with less to eat than what you paid for. "You soak beans," said the most frugal cook I know. "They don't soak you."

To cook beans, presoak them—with the exception of the smaller legumes, lentils and split peas, which needn't be soaked. Place them in a large pot with two to three times their volume of water and let them stand overnight or at least eight hours.

Alternatively, use the quick-soak method: bring the water to a boil and cook for one minute; turn off the heat, cover the pot, and allow the beans to stand for one to two hours. (This quick-soak method is supposed to reduce the likelihood that the beans will cause flatulence. Either way, discard the soaking water and cook them in fresh water.)

When you're ready to cook, bring the beans to a boil, then reduce the heat so you can cover the pot and let the beans simmer gently for the indicated amount of time.

If beans will be pressure-cooked, they do not require presoaking. Simply place them in the pressure cooker (three parts water to one part beans). Fill the cooker two-thirds full or less. Add one tablespoon of oil to prevent foaming. Cover and bring to pressure. Begin timing when the gauge rocks. After the time is up, cool the cooker until pressure is down before removing the lid.

Cooking Times for Beans

Type of Beans	*Stove Top (min.)*	*Pressure Cooker (min.)*
Black beans	90–120	22–25
Black-eyed peas	60–90	20
Chickpeas	120–180	40
Fava beans	120–180	40
Great Northern beans	90–120	25
Kidney beans	90–120	30
Lentils	30	N/A
Lima beans, small	90–120	20
Lima beans, large	120	30
Navy beans	120	30
Pinto beans	90–120	25
Soybeans	150–180	30–25
Split peas	30	N/A

Tofu 101

Do you have some friends that you really had to get to know before you liked them? Tofu can be like that. Once you get friendly with it, the odds are good that you'll be glad you did.

Tasteless on its own, tofu can take on the flavorings used with it to become a worthy pinch-hitter for such diverse and cholesterol-laden foods as ground beef, chicken, mayonnaise, cream cheese, sour cream, and eggs.

Made from soybeans, the richest in oil of all legumes, regular tofu weighs in at fifty-three percent fat per calorie. That's not low-fat when compared with other love-powered choices like bananas (three percent), cabbage (seven percent), and kidney beans (four percent). But when filling in for cream cheese (ninety-one percent fat), or hamburger or eggs (both sixty-five percent), there's a savings—not to mention that switching to tofu eliminates the other problems that come with using animal foods. Reduced-fat tofu is also available. White Wave makes one with a third less fat, and Mori-Nu makes one percent, low-fat silken tofu.

Tofu is economical, easy to digest, and if precipitated with calcium sulfate, a good source of calcium. (Read the label. I find that perhaps one-quarter of the tofu I see in the stores, maybe a little less, is calcium-cultured.) If you entertain guests a lot, or if you miss animal foods, or cook for a family that's resistant to change, tofu can make things easier.

By itself, tofu is like wet foam rubber, but you'd no more eat it by itself and expect fine dining than you would stare at a blank canvas and expect to see fine art. To become a Rembrandt with tofu, you first need to find it. Tofu is often in the produce department with the Asian vegetables. If you don't find it there, look in the dairy case where it's sometimes kept since it's so easily interchangeable with cottage, pot, farmer, feta, and ricotta cheeses. You can also locate tofu in aseptic packages so it needs no refrigeration.

Tofu is often labeled according to its consistency: "extra-firm," "firm," "soft," and "silken" (very soft). Firm can be used for everything; soft is used for dips, sauces, and spreads. It gets confusing because silken tofu (the softest) can be labeled "firm" and "extra-firm." Don't worry about it. Think of silken as soft, whatever the label says.

Tofu usually comes vacuum-packed in water, and if you have any left over after opening, you'll need to cover it with fresh water and change the water every two to three days.

Fresh tofu, when so cared for, will last seven to ten days in the refrigerator. (Unopened vacuum-packed tofu lasts quite a while when refrigerated; check the date on the container.) In aseptic cartons, silken tofu lasts indefinitely. These containers generally only contain ten ounces of tofu, so you don't need to worry about storing leftovers.

Try out these tasty, easy-to-make tofu fixings:

Salad dressing. Add to tofu in a blender a bit of lemon juice or cider vinegar, tamari (natural soy sauce), water as needed for the consistency you want, and whatever seasonings you fancy. My favorite is dried dillweed, but garlic and onion powder are always good, as is the spicy combo of curry and cumin.

Homemade tofu mayonnaise. Drain tofu. Place in a blender or food processor six ounces of tofu with two tablespoons of lemon juice, one tablespoon of oil, half a teaspoon of salt, a quarter of a teaspoon of white pepper, and purée. If desired, add seasonings like onions and garlic or pickles. (To lower the fat content, omit the oil.)

Sandwich spreads. Mix mashed tofu with chopped vegetables like carrots and celery. Thin with tofu mayonnaise for spreading consistency.

Burgers. Mix mashed tofu with chopped or grated vegetables (onions, peppers, mushrooms) and some sesame or ground sunflower seeds. Use flour to make the mixture stiff enough to form burgers. Season with salt, tamari, basil, cumin, garlic, onions. Bake or broil.

Tofu loaf. Use mashed tofu instead of ground beef in meat loaf.

Tofu steaks. Drain firm tofu. Slice in half-inch thicknesses. Coat with flour and spices. Bake until crisp. (This is especially good if you marinate the tofu first with a mixture of half water and half tamari.)

Soup. Cut drained tofu into little squares and use to replace chicken in chicken soup. Use a chicken-flavored vegetarian broth mix from a health food store for the base. Simmer long enough for tofu to pick up the flavor.

Pudding or "Yogurt." In a food processor, purée a block of tofu, about a tablespoon of agave nectar or maple syrup, a teaspoon of vanilla, and a dash of salt.

Adding carob powder or cocoa powder makes a chocolate-flavored pudding. (If you're a real yogurt fan, cultured soy yogurt is sold readymade in health food stores and many supermarkets. Stick with "plain" to keep the sugar content down. If you make yogurt yourself, that can be done with soymilk, too.)

The Granary

Solid, centering whole grains have been human dietary staples throughout recorded history. Although they're filling and replete with a wide range of minerals and B vitamins, a full cup averages less than two grams of fat. Most grains can be cooked, sprouted (wheat and rye sprout particularly well), ground into flour, made into pasta, cooked and sweetened as breakfast cereal, or cooked with savory seasonings as a side dish or entrée. When grains are sprouted, voilà!—they turn into vegetables.

For hot breakfast cereals, add extra water if not topping with milk or soymilk. Cook with dried fruit or a sweetener, perhaps overnight in a slow cooker, or sweeten with a little maple syrup or date sugar. For side dishes, use like rice to make a bed for black beans or stir-fried vegetables. Use grains as an entrée, such as rice pilaf, millet stuffing for squash or peppers, or couscous served with steamed vegetables.

For grains ground into flour, use whole-wheat flour for yeast breads, and whole-wheat pastry flour for quick breads, cookies, and pie crusts. Use cornmeal for corn bread, muffins, and Johnny cakes and buckwheat for pancakes. Try rye flours for specialty baking or as an alternative to wheat for people with allergies.

Whole-wheat spaghetti and lasagna noodles can be found in supermarkets. Health food stores stock not only these but also pastas made from corn, spelt, rice, quinoa, and buckwheat.

Whole grains can also be used in soups (barley is a natural here), in salads (think rice or pasta), or in desserts such as rice or bread pudding. Your supermarket can provide you with whole-wheat bread (be sure the wrapper says a hundred percent whole-wheat), whole-wheat pasta, brown rice, brown rice pilaf, wild rice, oatmeal, and whole-grain cold cereals. Health food stores have a vast array of whole grains as well as flours, pastas, and cereals made from them.

There are exotic grains to try like sticky-sweet amaranth and light, fluffy quinoa. And then there are the basics:

Brown rice. Long-grain brown rice cooks up in separate kernels to eat as is or for use in pilaf. Short-grain rice turns out sticky, which makes it good for croquettes and burgers or even pressed onto a pie plate as a fat-free crust for a tofu quiche or vegetable pie. Basmati is a gourmet rice from India with a nutty flavor and wonderful aroma. You can buy both brown and white basmati rice.

Buckwheat. Cook this like rice or as a hot breakfast cereal. Buckwheat (also called kasha) flour is fabulous for hotcakes.

Bulgur. Bulgur is cracked wheat, popular in Middle Eastern cooking, and the primary ingredient for tabbouleh, a wheat salad.

Corn. Although we don't tend to think of corn as a grain, we use cornmeal as such. Whole cornmeal—germ and bran included—is available at health food stores for use in hot cereal, bread, or polenta.

Millet. Tiny round grains that become puffy and delicate when cooked. Millet can be used as a cooked cereal, stuffing, the base for burgers, or a side dish.

Oats. You can cook whole oats (called groats), but oatmeal—even the quick-cooking kind—is a whole grain, too. Use for breakfast, in baking, or as the base for veggie burgers. (You can eat extracted oat bran if you want, but you may as well get the bran with the rest of the oat as a whole food.)

Scotch barley. This is whole-grain barley; the refined kind is called pearl barley. Use in soups or as an alternative to rice.

Wheat germ. This is the nutritious heart of the wheat kernel. It is therefore not a whole (intact) food, and it's fairly rich in oil. It is, however, a concentrated source of vegetable protein and vitamin E. Keep wheat germ stored in the refrigerator and buy it toasted, since raw wheat germ can go rancid very quickly. Wheat bran is sold separately, too, for dietary fiber, but the whole grain provides both the bran and the germ.

Whole wheat. Whole-wheat berries may be cooked or sprouted as well as ground into flour for bread or pasta. Couscous is a quick-cooking wheat product that has been pre-steamed. Most of the couscous available is refined, but even if you can't find the whole-grain variety, this quick-cooking, company-pleasing grain deserves a place in your pantry.

Wild rice. An elegant addition to a special meal, this North American native can dress up an ordinary rice dish or make an exquisite stuffing for winter squash.

All these whole grains keep well. Store them in jars with tight-fitting lids; keep the jars in a cool, dry place. Refrigerate whole-grain flours and cornmeal.

When it comes to cooking grains, Nava Atlas, author of *The Vegetarian Family Cookbook*, offers these simple suggestions: First, rinse the grains in a fine sieve (pre-steamed, rolled grains such as rolled oats don't require this). Toast them in a dry or lightly oiled skillet until the grains turn a shade darker and release a nutty aroma, then stir the grain into boiling water. Let it return to a boil and lower the heat; simmer, covered, until the water is absorbed. Don't stir while the grain is cooking. (Note: Rolled oats, bulgur, and couscous do not require simmering; just turn off the heat and allow the grain to sit for the specified time.) If grains are too chewy at the end of cooking time, add another half-cup of water for every cup of raw grain used; cover and simmer until water is absorbed.

Here are the cooking times for a few grains. These assume you're using two parts water to one part grain. Until you're used to whole grains, listen ahead of time to see if the simmering sound has stopped so you don't scorch a pot.

Grain Cooking Times

Grain	*Cooking Time (min.)*
Brown rice	45
Buckwheat (kasha)	20
Bulgur, cracked wheat	15
Millet	40
Quinoa	15
Rolled oats	10
Wheat berries	60–90

Fat Zappers

Our bodies don't require eggs or dairy foods or extracted oils, but for the kind of cooking we're used to, these foods seem essential. Vegetarian cookbooks can make you a masterful chef—or as close to that as you care to be—using no animal products and little oil. For the time being, try these culinary substitutions that really zap the fat out:

Eggs. Tofu Scrambler, a powdered product from Fantastic World foods, makes scrambled "eggs." In baking, substitute each egg with one teaspoon of commercial egg substitute and two tablespoons of water, or use one tablespoon of arrowroot powder, one tablespoon of soy flour, and two tablespoons of water; or blend two ounces of tofu with the liquid called for in the recipe. Half a large mashed banana works, too. In casseroles, burgers, and loaves, replace one egg with mashed potato, mashed avocado, or moistened bread crumbs or rolled oats.

Milk. Use soymilk (preferably low-fat), rice milk, or almond milk.

Cheese. In all honesty, you're not going to find a non-dairy cheese that's a dead ringer for your favorite sharp cheddar. There are, however, vegan cheeses at the health food store that are quite tasty to all but the cheese connoisseur. (Their fat content is comparable to dairy cheese but without the cholesterol.) Substitute mashed soft tofu for ricotta or feta in recipes, or look for the commercial soy feta at natural food stores—delicious.

Nutritional yeast or tahini (sesame butter) can substitute for Parmesan on pasta, or get soy Parmesan (or a raw alternative, Parma!) at health food stores. For cream cheese, use firm tofu blended with salt, dill, and lime juice to taste, or purchase vegan cream cheese—high in fat but so close in taste and texture to the genuine article I've fooled cream-cheese-and-bagel people with it many times. A great collection of recipes for those who think this cheese thing could be a deal-breaker is *The Ultimate Uncheese Cookbook* by Joanne Stepaniak.

Shortening. In baking, substitute natural applesauce or prune purée (prune baby food works great) for the oil, butter, or shortening you'd otherwise use. You can also leave out up to one-third of the fat called for in the recipe without affecting the flavor, and puréed tofu can fill in for two-thirds of the remaining butter or oil.

Kitchen Ecology

. . . .

Simply eating a plant-based diet takes pressure off the Earth. In doing so, for example, you save acres of trees every year and, in not supporting the meat industry, you take your dollars away from a business that contributes greatly to greenhouse gases. There are additional simple practices that you can undertake to lighten the planet's burden even more:

Use cloth or string bags when you shop. If you've ever lived outside the United States, you already know that this is a natural and pleasant way to shop. If you're without your cloth bags, paper is a slightly better choice than plastic. Either way, reuse and then recycle them.

Buy in bulk when you can. Health food stores and co-ops often offer whole grains, flours, nuts, seeds, dried fruit, olive oil, maple syrup, and even household cleaning products in bulk, allowing you to use your own refillable containers. When you have a choice, choose the product with the least packaging.

Store foods in jars you've saved or in other reusable containers. This will cut down on your use of plastic wrap and foil. You can also try cellulose storage bags made from plant fiber.

Save energy. You can do this by including lots of raw foods in your diet and by not cooking at the highest heat setting. Only run your dishwasher when it's full. When it's time to by a new appliance, look for one with an Energy Star rating.

Compost your food scraps. This actually turns your garbage into rich soil that can be used in a garden or simply donated back to the earth. It's easier than you think.

Insist on real dishes. Stay out of fast-food places with their throwaway accoutrements. Keep a mug at the office and have a refillable covered container to take to the coffee bar or bring along in your car. Suggest a switch to washable cups at your church and club groups. If you must go with a disposable once in a while, OK; but never, ever use Styrofoam: that cup will be intact in a landfill *2,000* years from now. Get yourself a picnic basket stocked with casual dishes so you won't use paper. Collect funky mismatched plates and silverware at tag sales so you can serve a crowd without disposables. And when you go for Chinese, forego the toss-away chopsticks. (Chopsticks are fun and some weight-loss experts recommend them for slowing down a meal. For the sake of the planet, just bring your own. You can even find foldable chopsticks online.)

Use cloth napkins. To make this practical, you won't want all your napkins lace-edged or made of heavy linen that needs to be ironed. You can even buy cotton or cotton/polyester bandannas, reasonably

---

Kitchen Ecology (*continued*)

. . . .

priced at camping equipment stores. One napkin a week per family member may be enough, but keep plenty on hand for guests, spills, and messy meals.

Allow clean dishes to air-dry. By doing so, you'll avoid the energy drain of your dishwasher's drying cycle. And whether you do your dishes by machine or with a pair of rubber gloves, use a detergent that's environmentally sound and tested without the use of animals.

Every concerned and loving action you take shows the love-empowerment working in your life. Using a cloth bag instead of plastic is like making yourself a couple of baked potatoes instead of tearing into a bag of chips. Both show you care, and it's pretty difficult to practice genuine caring and addictive behavior at the same time.

Salad dressings. Blend vegetables and herbs with tomato and lemon juice, or cut oil in conventional recipes by half and substitute tomato juice or blended tofu. Also, try blending a small amount of nuts, seeds, or avocado with carrot, celery, or tomato juice—or with water, lemon, and savory seasonings to taste. Another option is to squeeze fresh lime juice onto a salad to allow the taste of the vegetables to come through. Fresh lime or lemon juice and seasoned salt or an herbal spice blend makes for a sophisticated salad.

Oil. Use non-stick cookware to eliminate or cut down on oil (high-quality cookware with tight-fitting lids retains steam from vegetables, minimizing the amount of oil and other liquids required). Also, spray-coat pans instead of pouring on oil, or use other liquids such as water, tomato juice, cooking sherry, apple juice, tamari (the reduced-fat kind works best for cooking), vegetable broth, or an oil/water combination (one tablespoon of oil to a third of a cup of water).

Good Food Gadgets

You don't need a kitchen filled with paraphernalia to create meals your body will truly appreciate. The important utensils will be some nice wooden spoons for stirring; a big bowl or two for mixing and for salads; a sharp chef's knife and a paring knife; a couple of pieces of good, non-aluminum cookware with lids; a vegetable steamer; and either a blender or a food processor for making spreads, sauces, smoothies, cream soups, and the like.

Among the following good food gadgets, you'll find some you already own and some you may want to invest in. None is indispensable.

Blender. Ideal for shakes, smoothies, salad dressings, and sauces. Some natural-food folk swear by the high-powered Vita-Mix and K-Tec brands. My plain old blender does the job.

Citrus juicer. Inexpensive models, either manual or electric, are found in discount, department, and cookware stores. Fresh grapefruit, orange, and tangerine juices are exquisite.

Double boiler. Has two pots; one holds boiling water, the other holds the food. Cooks gently—excellent for preparing grains such as millet or for reheating leftovers.

Food processor. Shreds, chops, mixes, and kneads. Helpful for making salads, dips, and purées.

Hot-air popcorn popper. For fat-free popcorn that you can season yourself with tamari, nutritional yeast (for cheesy taste), or a dash of ground pepper.

Non-stick cookware. Cut down on oil use by buying at least one high-quality, non-stick pan. Get one with a lengthy guarantee against chipping of the coating. It's also good to look for non-stick cookware that doesn't require the use of special utensils: unless you live alone, someone is bound to use the wrong spatula. I like Millennium from Farberware. (Not all your cookware has to be non-stick. Have at least one piece—a Dutch oven or soup pot perhaps—in cast iron to maximize your iron absorption.)

Rice cooker. This is a great boon for cooking perfect rice and for steaming vegetables. Plug it in and don't worry.

Pressure cooker. Popular in the 1950s, pressure cookers are back in more sophisticated models. Pressure-cooking is a real time-saver when beans are on the menu.

Salad spinner. This nifty contraption in cookware departments and gourmet shops will spin-dry salad greens in a jiffy.

Slow cooker. Let a slow cooker simmer up a one-pot dinner (soup, stew, chili, or homemade grain pilaf) while you're away for the day.

Sprouter. If you'd like to grow sprouts in a more sophisticated manner than the cheesecloth and jar technique (see "Sprout Farming" earlier in this chapter) there are perforated plastic trays, special bamboo bags, and a variety of other inventions for growing your sprout garden. Look for these at health food stores or online.

Vegetable juicer. Try a juicer with centrifugal force—it works great for extracting juices from carrots, greens, and all kinds of fruit. If you invest in a full-service juicer such as the Champion or the Green Star, you'll also be able to make soft-serve fruit-based frozen desserts and fresh nut butters. Look for these in health food stores and online.

Vegetable steamer. You can get the vitamins and great taste that you'd otherwise miss in cooked vegetables by buying a stainless steel vegetable steaming rack for just a few dollars. Place it over boiling water in a pot with a tight-fitting lid. Put the vegetables on top and enjoy them a few minutes later.

Wok. You can stir-fry in a large skillet, but a wok—an electric wok or one that you put on the stove—invites the frequent use of this healthful style of cooking. Look into a non-stick wok to keep oil use to a minimum.

You'll notice that I didn't mention microwaves. It's true that they save time and energy, and they can be a real help in cooking without added fats. If you already have one, you probably love it, so use it in good health. I don't recommend microwaves, however, because I don't think that microwaved food tastes as good as food cooked conventionally. As a practicing binge eater, I ate food no matter how it tasted. I don't have to do that today. Now I can have the best even if it means waiting for it.

Also, I believe that too much dependence upon microwaving—as well as on fast-food restaurants—can impede a food addict's recovery. Both provide food lickety-split—the ideal setup for a binge. When you cook beans and grains the old-fashioned way, taking your time is a given. When you're eating raw fruits and vegetables, there's no time spent fixing them, but plenty of time goes into chewing. Either way, a slow-down factor is built in.

Also of value is seeing that your kitchen is a place that makes you smile. If yours is filled with unhappy memories of sneaking leftovers and midnight refrigerator raids, christen it as a new place, a friendly location supportive of your true needs. Hang up a picture that you treasure or quotations that mean something to you. You may want to treat yourself to new tableware. When I had a set of pottery dishes made that I'd designed myself, I felt special. A bit of that feeling has stayed with each plate and bowl and mug. Every meal with these dishes feels like a special occasion, even though the set cost no more than ordinary stoneware.

Start with small things: Delight in your dishes or your herb plants or the inspirational needlework saying on the wall. You'll soon delight as well in how your eating has changed. It's all connected.

CHAPTER NINE

LOVE-POWERED LIVING

A love-powered life is a life of love and power. It doesn't come from the personal ego—defined, someone told me, as "edging God out"—but from the unlimited power of love. When we talk about the power that heats houses and runs factories, the synonym we use for it is energy. Adopting love-powered principles, spiritually and physically, brings abundant energy into our lives. For one thing, there's more energy available from eating this way. Unrefined carbohydrates are known for fueling endurance athletes. And we can better take advantage of this greater energy because of the changes that have taken place in our thoughts and attitudes.

There are no rigid rules for living a love-based rather than a fear-based life. In general, though, this new way of relating to yourself and your world can be defined by the ABCs: it's Addiction-free, Balanced, and Compassionate.

Addiction-free. Spiritual renewal makes freedom from addiction possible. Sensible choices on the physical level are supportive of this. With daily dedication to your new way of life, you can expect not only freedom from the food fix but freedom from other imbalances that have held you back.

Balance. True balance comes about when generous portions of love and power are expressed harmoniously in a person's life. I think of it as working like this:

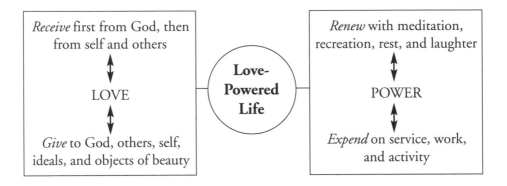

In practice, giving and receiving love become the same thing. Love can't be stored up like grain in a silo or coins in a jar, so the love you get must go out again. You become a conduit rather than a container. The more love you give, the more you're able to channel. It's the ultimate in recycling. Energy operates similarly. You renew your supply in quiet times with your Higher Power, and with rest, sleep, and having fun. Work that you love, exuberant activity, and doing some good in the world can also give energy back to you.

Compassion. Love and energy—giving and receiving, expending and renewing—enable lives to work. Lives that work best also reveal compassion. Compassion is the keynote of love-powered eating and compassion—although interpreted in different ways—is central to any viable spirituality. The word's literal meaning is "to feel with." You can "feel with" another because you've been hurt yourself and can empathize, or because you've had compassion shown to you and you know how to pass it on.

The Balance of Healthful Living

There are many ways in which balance makes itself evident in a life—among them are harmonious relationships, productive work, and responsible financial dealings. But balance also means taking good care of yourself physically and recognizing that food addiction is adept at robbing its victims of the will to care for themselves. As you progress in appreciating yourself, you'll develop enough self-love to want to care for yourself and enough energy to actually do it. The self-care then creates more energy.

At the heart of self-care are some specific laws of life that lead to health and happiness. When they're ignored or denied, we get the opposite results. These important laws include: eating pure food that enhances physical wellbeing; doing regular, vigorous exercise; getting plenty of rest and sleep; breathing fresh air; drinking pure water; establishing a respectful relationship with the sun; and managing stress levels by developing peace of mind and emotional poise.

I used to think that if a person were spiritual enough, the physical self wouldn't matter. Now I see "spiritual" and "physical" as concentric circles, or colors in a rainbow, one fading into the next. The fact that there are natural laws to help us get more joy out of life is as close to a gift from God as anything I know of.

When I was an active food addict, taking care of myself was near the bottom of my priority list. At times I slide back into some of my old ways, but the natural laws are always there for my benefit and yours. Maybe I didn't get enough sleep the previous night or maybe I was traveling and used that as an excuse to avoid exercise for five days straight. I can take a nap now. I can exercise today. So can you. And these healthy habits are self-propagating. Once you make room for them in your life, things don't seem right without them.

Love Yourself with Activity

Exercise is good for the body and even better for the spirit. Long before you observe that an increase in your activity level has blessed you with firmer muscles, greater stamina, and a more efficient metabolic rate, you'll notice a heightened sense of wellbeing and self-worth. I know that this is true even though I have a long history of detesting almost any endeavor capable of producing perspiration. In recent years, I've come to appreciate how good moving my body can make me feel. Sometimes I love it; sometimes I just go through the motions. When I start to truly dislike the exercise I'm doing, I know it's time to change it. That's because the body doesn't exercise alone; the mind comes along, too, and it also needs to enjoy itself.

It's not always easy because even the vocabulary that refers to physical activity makes it seem like chain-gang labor. *Exercise* sounds like *exertion*; people can be hospitalized for that. A *workout* doesn't sound like a great time either. My friend Dr. Douglas Graham, surely one of the fittest people I know, tells his patients, "I don't want you to work out. You work all day. In your free time I expect you to play."

Someone who's already fit like Dr. Graham might play as he does: jumping on a trampoline in the backyard, hiking in the woods of Maine, skiing in Colorado, swimming in the Gulf of Mexico, taking hundred-mile bike trips, or maneuvering through town on in-line skates with the agility of a carefree school kid on the first day of summer vacation. People who've been battling with their bodies for years, however, don't automatically equate exercise with play or pleasure. "Workout" seems like a most appropriate term, because hard exercise taken too soon can feel like work, drudgery even.

Most of us who were overweight as children have horrible memories about sports and athletics. We were chosen last for teams and grudgingly at that. We were called names by our classmates and chided by our gym teachers, and we experienced real suffering doing what everyone else apparently regarded as fun. We rubbed sores on our thighs when we tried to run. Our throats burned as we gasped for air, hoping to keep up in the sprint or make it to the bases. And the emotional pain of being seen in a swimsuit or showering after gym class was as acute as any physical discomfort.

Specific, conscious memories can fade, but those painful feelings attach themselves in our minds to the entire realm of exercise and participatory sports. It's no wonder that even after we're grown up (and even if we slim down) many of us regard exercise as a threat. People who were not heavy in childhood but gained extra weight later can have another problem. They remember how good it once felt to run and jump and dance. Thinking that they can't do these things now makes them feel sad and old when decades of promise still lie before them.

But you *can* move your body and enjoy doing it. Whether you were heavy as a child or not, regardless of your current weight or age, you'll be a happier as well as a fitter person when you start to use your muscles regularly and pleasurably. Remember that we're talking about a loving approach to diet and to life. A "no pain, no gain" philosophy doesn't fit here; taking it slow is not only advisable, it's mandatory.

For exercise to do for you all that it can, it has to become an integral part of your life. It's not to be used like some willpower diet until you get to some arbitrary number on a scale. And it's not to be put off until after you're thin, after they run a special at the health club, or after you get around to putting air in your bicycle tires. You do it today because your body is a living organism that craves movement. Look at toddlers and puppies: the urge to be active is innate. If you think that urge in you is dead, it isn't. It's only sleeping. Don't try to jolt it awake with fifty pushups and a five-mile run. Nudge it gently.

If you're over forty, overweight, or have health problems requiring a special exercise regimen (diabetes, high blood pressure, heart disease, and arthritis are among these), by all means work out your fitness program with a knowledgeable professional. In any case, begin slowly. This is not just because it's easier on your heart and your joints to build up gradually but also because if you don't love what you're doing, you're likely to leave it. Sporadic exercise—a week here, a weekend there, a long layoff, then a ski trip—does almost nothing for a body and is an open invitation to injury.

Ideally, you exercise because you love both yourself and the activity. It's not necessary that you be a distance runner, a belly dancer, or a power lifter. What's necessary for a fit and healthy life is that you be active enough for your body to function optimally. The general rule for accomplishing this is a minimum of thirty minutes of aerobic exercise four to six times a week. Aerobic (oxygen-utilizing) exercises are those that can be done for prolonged periods—such as walking, running, swimming, skating, cycling, rowing, or dancing. This type of exercise is believed to be of particular benefit to the heart and circulatory system, to revive a sluggish metabolism, and to help normalize an unreasonable appetite.

Aerobic activity is not the only sort of useful motion that exists, however. The luxurious limbering and stretching of yoga and modern dance promote youthful flexibility, while weight training sculpts a body to its best and provides it with more lean tissue. Lean tissue is a metabolism booster. These three activities—aerobics (cardio), stretching, and resistance exercise (weight training)—work together to create the kind of fitness you deserve and the kind of body you've dreamed of.

Customize your program. If you're a loner, you may want to invest in a stationary bike or a treadmill. If you love the outdoors, you'll probably prefer to jog or cycle whenever the weather permits and schedule some enjoyable backup activity when it doesn't. If you're gregarious, you'll like taking classes or belonging to a gym. Don't expect your basic personality to change to fit your exercise plan: it won't.

I myself live with a state-of-the-art treadmill. Am I using it? Not on your life. I'm at my desk communicating with you. I'm a communicator, one of the gregarious types. When I'm at the health club, I exercise (and communicate) energetically; if I had to exercise at home by myself, I'd probably be suffering from advanced muscle atrophy. Know yourself, but don't take so much time figuring out what kind of exercise you might like that you never get around to exercise at all. Join a gym, join the Y, enroll in a class, and then show up. Make it a habit. For most people, working out every morning with one rest day is the best system since it makes exercise a regular habit without three-or-four-day layoffs that can become three or four weeks.

Some of the ways you may wish to meet your inborn need for activity are:

Walking. Where do you like to walk? Through the woods? Along country roads? I love to walk in cities. From my point of view, the best part of being in New York City or Chicago or San Francisco is walking all over, feeding pigeons, looking in shop windows, exploring parks and cathedrals, and taking in the sights and sounds and energy of the city. When walking is your activity of choice, you can do it anywhere, and the only equipment it takes is a pair of sturdy, well-fitting walking shoes. If you don't like the idea of exercise, see your walking as simply taking a walk. My friend Robin calls people she knows and asks if they would like to walk with her, the way we would more often ask someone out for a drink or a meal. It's a really charming invitation. Or walk alone. Then you can vary your pace to suit yourself. Your walking may evolve into a nicely paced run. On alternating days when you aren't looking for a bona fide aerobic workout, you may forgo speeding things up in favor of slowing them down. Then you can treat yourself to the serenity of meditative walking.

Swimming. The problem with swimming is the bathing suit. The real difficulty there lies not so much in the suits or how we look in them but how we think that

Exercise Obsession

. . . .

Obsessive exercise is any fitness program that interferes with your life as a whole. New exercisers are often overzealous, but they soon become more moderate. Obsessive exercise, however, is not self-correcting. Like other addictions, it's progressive.

Knowing whether you're exercising obsessively or just enthusiastically can be a tough call. A person who works out six times a week but can skip a day without regret is probably not obsessed with exercise. But another person exercising six days a week may rigidly stick to that workout schedule even when it means exacerbating an injury, rescheduling important business appointments, or missing her child's first softball game of the season. That's interfering with life.

If you're accustomed to exercising regularly, you feel a letdown without it. Your body and mind get used to steady doses of endorphins, the feel-good chemicals that your system produces in response to vigorous activity. Your muscles become accustomed to exercising daily (or four times a week, or whatever your schedule is). And if you're doing exercise that you really like, you look forward to it as a form of recreation as well. All these motivators are good because they make it easier to incorporate exercise into your life.

Obsessive exercise, however, isn't motivated by wanting to feel good, having eager muscles, or enjoying recreation. It comes from believing that your worth is dependent upon how much you exercise and how buff you become. Many of us, particularly if we've been fat or thought we were, measure our worth with a scale, skin-fold calipers, and a tape around the waist. The size, shape, and firmness of our bodies become indicators of our value as human beings. If we believe this, we no longer choose to exercise, we're forced to. The exercise is healthy, but the motivation isn't. When we're pushed to exert ourselves beyond a reasonable point, the physical activity itself can become detrimental.

Here are some questions to ask yourself if you think that you may be an obsessive exerciser.

- Do I exercise when I'm injured or sick?

- Do I exercise when it means skimping on sleep?

- Do I cancel social or professional plans in order to exercise?

- Do I skip meals to exercise (with or without compulsively eating later to compensate)?

- Do I feel guilty when I miss a workout?

Exercise Obsession (*continued*)

. . . .

- Do I keep close track of the results that exercise is having on my body by weighing and measuring myself persistently?

- Do I yo-yo from exercising a lot (seven to fifteen or more hours a week) to not at all?

- Do I exercise to make up for overeating?

If you answered affirmatively to two or more of these questions, you may be exercise-obsessive. If you answered the last question affirmatively, you could be exercising to rationalize binge eating. This is particularly dangerous because using exercise as an excuse to binge makes physical activity part of your food (and/or dieting) addiction. Juggling overeating (and/or undereating) with compulsive exercise is a trying performance. The inner changes that arrest food addiction can do the same with exercise addiction. You should also:

Dedicate yourself to wellness, not thinness. When overall wellness is your goal, a balanced life is more important than rapid weight loss or flattening your abdomen in fourteen days.

Guard against thinking of exercise in terms of calories utilized. If you find yourself rationalizing extra food or a food you know to be harmful by telling yourself, "I'll take an extra cardio class this week," you're on shaky ground. Use your spiritual principles and your support group to set your thinking straight.

Set a reasonable schedule for exercise and stay with that. Three days a week should be the bare minimum, six the maximum. (Your body needs one day a week to rest.)

Respect your body's current needs. The body requires regular exercise, but circumstances can make other needs a priority. If you're in the acute stage of an illness, even if it's just a cold, you need rest, not exercise. If you're injured, you need to lay off or change the kind of exercise you do (switch from running to swimming, for example) until you've healed.

Make exercise a part of your life as a whole. Make some of your activity part of your family life (a Saturday morning bike ride, walking with your spouse, running with the dog) or your social activities (joining a folk dance club or a hiking group). Some exercise can also be incidental like walking to the grocery store or cycling to the office. When your exercise has more meaning than what it's doing for your hips, obsession is less apt to take over.

Consider your commitment to exercise a long-term one. When you really believe that you'll stay active for life, it's not threatening to go easy or take a day off when you need to.

Exercise Obsession (*continued*)

. . . .

Use some of your exercise time for less rigorous activities such as restorative yoga, tai chi, a delicious stretch class, or meditative walking. Beyond the aerobic conditioning your heart deserves and the weight training needed by your muscles and bones, you can choose from a variety of gentler activities. If you're obsessive about exercise, you may rail against the milder pursuits that don't seem to burn enough calories to be worth your time. They will, however, slow you down so you can actually experience your body—an experience impaired by both compulsive eating and compulsive exercise.

Please note that purging (vomiting), laxative abuse, *and* compulsive exercise are bulimic behaviors, manipulative methods enabling a person to eat for a fix without the natural consequence of gaining weight. If you purge or abuse laxatives, you're a prime candidate for exercise obsession, too. Your recovery may require growing beyond these cover-up activities before your eating moderates on a consistent basis. Trust the process to deal with first things first, and get whatever help (be it medical, psychological, or spiritual) that you need to get these dangerous and demoralizing *dis ease* patterns out of your life for good.

we ought to look in them. Self-acceptance may never have a tougher test than the swimsuit competition—the one in which the beautiful reality that you are today is challenged by advertising's persuasive image of how a body is supposed to look. Your growth in self-love will help you win in that internal swimsuit competition, and your new lifestyle will bring your body to its ideal state of health and fitness. Swimming—suit and all—can be part of that.

When you swim, you feel light. Movements that would be labored if not impossible on land can be almost effortless. Swimming is a cardiovascular activity, yet it's also relaxing and conducive to contemplation. One winter I belonged to a health club equipped with an indoor/outdoor pool. I went in the mornings before work and felt incredibly accomplished when I showed up at the office knowing that I'd been swimming while snow fell all around me. If you plan to swim, be sure that the pool you choose has an atmosphere that's really pleasing to you. If the hours there aren't convenient, if the water is too cold, or, for that matter, the staff is too cold, look elsewhere.

One caveat: unless you have access to a lake, ocean, saltwater pool or one that's purified by some means other than chlorination, you probably shouldn't be swimming more than once or twice a week. For all the benefits of the activity, doing it in a heavily chlorinated pool may not be wise. Your skin is a living, breathing organ that absorbs some of what it's exposed to. This doesn't mean you should stop swimming. Simply cross-train so you're not swimming in chlorine every day.

Cycling. Bicycling appeals to my practical nature since it can be efficient transportation as well as aerobic exercise. If you can possibly use a bike for some of your commuting needs, I can almost guarantee that your life will change for the better in ways you might never have imagined. If you bike to work, your status in the company will improve even before your next promotion. That's because people are awed when someone actually demonstrates self-sufficiency, and getting to the job via person-power is self-sufficiency of the highest order. My fondest memory as a pedaling commuter is whizzing past the bus I'd otherwise have taken every morning. Of course, the same hill that enabled me to fly past a bus on my morning route had me huffing and puffing in the evening. It was worth it.

Biking is excellent for the not-yet-in-shape because you can pace it to your fitness level from short trips on flat land to touring the Rockies. It helps to have a comfortable bicycle. The balloon-tire single-speed bike in the garage can provide you with a workout, but a bike with gears lets you compensate for hills and feel less fatigued.

Some day you may want to race or enter a triathlon or get into mountain biking. Then again, you may prefer to pedal a stationary bike in your own family room while you watch a sitcom on TV. You get what you're after either way.

Dance exercise classes. If you always wanted to be in a Broadway chorus line you'll love dance exercise classes. They provide the opportunity for anyone to dance, regardless of her number of left feet. (I say "her" because these classes are overwhelmingly female, but men who summon the nerve to try it have a really good time. And, as you may imagine, the two or three men in a class of women are very popular.) They're always coming up with a new twist on the decades-old concept of "aerobic dance," but the fact is, dance was aerobic (i.e., using oxygen) both before that word was coined and now that it sounds dated. You can find hip-hop, Latin, musical theater, and even pole-dancing classes to spice things up.

My preference is for low-impact classes to minimize stress on the joints. Just because it's called low-impact, however, doesn't mean that a class is low-intensity. It can be quite intense and call for a well-developed state of fitness to be fun or, for that matter, effective. If a session is too difficult, it won't even be aerobic for you: You'll over-exert and your heart rate will go beyond the aerobic training range—the point at which you're breathing hard enough to know that you're exercising, but not so hard that you can't comfortably carry on a conversation. Don't sign up for any classes you can't try out first; if a class is too tough and the instructor won't help you tone it down, find another.

Sometimes health clubs offer classes geared to beginners or senior citizens. I took a daily seniors' class when I was still in my thirties because it was the only one that fit my schedule. Along with weight training, that class put me at my highest level of fitness ever. It was easy enough to be fun; I enjoyed it, so I rarely missed a session. The teachers were friendly and down-to-earth; the participants encouraged each other. These are important qualities for you to look for in a cardio-dance program. Teachers should also be certified to teach aerobics and the facilities should accommodate this kind of class, with enough room for every student and a shock-absorbent floor to protect your knees and ankles as you exercise. Finally, the music needs to make you happy. If you like the music, chances are you'll stick with the class—and you'll hum a lot the rest of the time.

Weight training. Working with weights can make profound changes in how your body looks in a short time. Even more meaningful is how differently people start to regard themselves when they've been involved with weight training for a while. Instead of feeling weak or routinely taking the victim's role, a person who trains with weights notices a feeling of competence and confidence after only a few weeks. Strong people tend to feel strong, inside and out. You can set up a home gym, but a well-equipped club can provide you with safety, instruction, and moral support. Working with a personal trainer who really cares about your progress can make up for all the unkind gym teachers you ever had. Verbal support like, "One more lift:

I know you can do it" can work wonders, not just for your triceps but for your sense of self.

Weight training reshapes and, literally, re-creates your body. It's the first step in any anti-aging program in that it arrests much of the loss of muscle mass that starts in our thirties and goes crazy after menopause. With more muscle, your metabolism is higher so you burn more calories even at rest. And weight training builds bone as well as muscle, helping ensure mobility and independence in your later years.

Ideally, you'll either do full-body weight training two or three times a week with one or two rest days in between, or work out six times a week alternating upper and lower body workouts. (You can work your abs daily. Thought you'd like to know!)

Yoga. If you don't love your body yet, yoga can help you get to that point silently and surely. Hatha (physical) yoga—postures and breathing techniques—is thousands of years old. It comes from the Indian subcontinent, but its benefits aren't confined to a single country or belief system. The slow movements of traditional yoga, coupled with controlled breathing, result in a calming of the body and mind. Yoga develops flexibility of the entire body, particularly the spine, and is believed to have various therapeutic applications.

Yoga was the first step I took in learning to love and care for myself. It put me in touch with my body. I'd long tried to forget that I had a body since I always judged it as being fat or flabby or in some other way not measuring up. In yoga, I began to experience my body in a non-threatening environment. The first thing I noticed was that I did have some natural flexibility. My self-image was then able to incorporate for the first time a positive trait that didn't have to do with being intelligent or having a good personality, but one that belonged to my physical self. I also found my yoga teachers to be kind and patient. I remember one teacher saying, "Don't worry about changing your diet. Allow your spirituality to grow and that will change your diet." She turned out to be right.

If you're interested in yoga, visit a class and get a sense of it. Instructors of traditional hatha yoga are adept at the slow, calming style of this ancient discipline. There are other styles of yoga that are more rigorous, challenging, and invigorating. All styles are good. The key to knowing the right one for you is that you feel better when you leave yoga class than when you arrived. Just as you'll need a mat to protect your back when you practice, your class should have an atmosphere that's like a cushion. After all, you're loving yourself to thinness, so you may as well love yourself to fitness, too.

Love Yourself with Rest

Our society doesn't respect rest and sleep. Resting is seen as laziness and sleep as a wasteful, albeit unavoidable, time expenditure. We reluctantly fit them in because we'd collapse if we didn't. Pushing ourselves, even with stimulants like caffeine, is the accepted way of things. Whether the goal is the honor roll or the executive suite, we give our work all we've got. That's fine up to a point, until we realize that "all we've got" is, physically, all we have. What we're talking about—this intangible substance that propels us—is vital energy: the yogis' *prana*. Whatever we call it, it has to be regularly replenished. The natural way to do that is with adequate rest and sleep. And here's an all-points bulletin for you: recent research has shown that lack of sleep can keep people fat. It distorts metabolism and can cause a craving for sweets.

Agreeing, then, that sleep is necessary: How much do you need? Whatever is enough for you to feel good. Most adults require at least seven hours of sleep per night. One way to find out what's right for you is to stop using an alarm clock. Try this on the weekends first so you won't be afraid of being late for work and wake up at three AM wondering if you've overslept. After you've done this for a while, you'll discover that you have an exceedingly efficient internal clock. When you awaken to it, you'll be refreshed. Even confirmed night people become much more tolerant of mornings when the clock radio is silenced and the internal clock takes over. (Don't worry about missing music in the morning: Do this and you'll sing.)

If you've had trouble sleeping, many of the lifestyle changes recommended in this book may be helpful. People who've considered themselves chronic insomniacs have found that simply cutting out caffeine, not just in the evening but all the time, solves the problem. Exercise is also valuable. The body strives for balance (the fancy word for that physiological balance is *homeostasis*), so exercise naturally invites rest and sleep as its balancers. Meditation, too, produces the deep relaxation that encourages peaceful sleep.

Sleep isn't the only kind of rest we need, however. We're supposed to rest whenever our bodies give us "tired signals." We've misinterpreted these signals in all sorts of ways. For most food addicts, tired feels like hungry. The message can also reach our brain sounding like, "It's time for a cup of coffee," "Work harder, lazy!" or "Everything is irritating me and I'm about to explode." The next time you get any of those messages in the midst of a busy day, take a minute to examine them. Behind the hunger or the caffeine craving or the irritation might just be your body asking for a catnap, a walk outdoors, a brief conversation with another person, or just a switch from answering e-mail to returning a call.

When you have sizable chunks of rest time, be sure that your rest is really restful. Watching the news or a murder mystery on television isn't an athletic event, but it's not resting either. You can rest with a book, but you can rest more fully while lying in a hammock watching the clouds. You can rest in a reclining chair listening to soothing music. You can rest by daydreaming, contemplating, or unwinding in a bath scented with lavender or juniper. Massage can also be sublimely restful. Honor your uniqueness by discovering those restful pursuits that make you say "Ahh."

Love Yourself with Fresh Air

Take a nice, deep breath. It feels good, doesn't it? Do it again and really blow the air out on the exhalation. It's a great sensation, both relaxing and energizing at the same time. Our breath is our lifeline, although we seldom give it any conscious attention. We don't have complete control over the *quality* of the air we breathe, but there are some actions we can take to breathe a little easier.

If you smoke, stop. Certainly this is a tall order because nicotine addiction is a powerful one. Whether you want to deal with your overeating or your smoking first, or whether you want to make both of those changes simultaneously, is up to you. Smoking is generally regarded as a more rapid form of suicide than binge eating, but to get all the life you're entitled to, get rid of both. Don't worry about eating more when you quit smoking. You're committed to loving and caring for yourself—your *whole* self. As long as you cling to any crutch to stay thin, especially a potentially fatal crutch like cigarettes, you won't know the freedom of total recovery.

Get the help you need to quit from your doctor and other resources. The American Cancer Society and the American Lung Association both have programs to help smokers become ex-smokers. Seventh Day Adventist churches and the hospitals affiliated with them also offer effective smoking-cessation programs. (Their suggestions include cutting out red meat and caffeine to lessen the craving for nicotine; so you, as a love-powered eater, would be ahead of the game.) The most important thing is that you don't give up.

If you don't smoke, don't breathe someone else's. Many cities and states have banned smoking in public places. When you're somewhere that allows it, claim some pollution-free space as best you can. I've never been a smoker, but it used to be that when a hostess at a restaurant asked, "Smoking or nonsmoking?" I'd say, "It doesn't matter." That translates as "I don't matter." But I do, and you matter just as much. You have rights; stand up for them. This is especially true in your own home. If no one in your family smokes, no one who visits should get to smoke. Your home may not be a castle, but it doesn't have to smell like a pool hall either.

On other airy matters:

Open windows, especially at night. We go so nonchalantly from central heating to central air-conditioning that we forget there's another kind of air—the fresh kind. Letting some in will revive your spirits and having fresh air circulating in your bedroom at night can become a positive habit you'll always keep. Expect your quality of sleep to improve once you try this. (If it's winter, just open a window a little and use an extra blanket.)

Give your household air a pollution check. Look in the Yellow Pages under "Environmental Services" or "Air Pollution Control" to find a company that can inform you about your indoor air quality. They'll check for pollutants such as radon (airborne particles of radium from decaying rock that are believed to cause lung cancer), formaldehyde (a suspected carcinogen that can come from carpets, paneling, and formaldehyde-foam insulation), and carbon monoxide as a combustion byproduct of fuels, as well as for dusts and molds that can aggravate allergies. If problems are found, there are ways (other than moving) to remedy them. Getting your air ducts cleaned every couple of years is a good idea, too.

Don't be a domestic polluter. Improve your home's air quality by using environmentally sound household cleaners, commercial or homemade, in place of harsh chemicals. Fumes from these (whether you can smell them much or not) end up in the air you breathe. (Just as using strong chemicals can decrease your air quality, having houseplants around can increase it by providing additional oxygen.)

Do what you can to curb pollution in your community. Plant trees. Support clean air legislation. Become involved in local pollution-control campaigns or back the people who are involved.

And treat yourself to gourmet air whenever possible. Gourmet air is the best there is—the sort you'll find in the mountains, in the woods, and at the shore. Nature's most beautiful spots are also first-rate air purifiers.

Love Yourself with Water

You can love yourself with water externally and internally. We take baths and showers for granted, but have you noticed lately that it feels terrific to get clean? A shower is an invigorating experience; a bath is relaxing. Either one can be made special by using products that smell and feel good. There's no reason why men as well as women can't treat themselves to sumptuous scents. The products that incorporate aromatherapy—oils that not only smell wonderful but are believed to have subtle, therapeutic effects on the mind and body—aren't gender-exclusive.

Baths call for a lot more water than showers do. If you're going to take a bath, make it worth the water. Set aside enough time to really enjoy the process. Turn off the ringer on your phones so your thoughts won't turn from your relaxing bath to "Who could that be?" (I've left a hot, fragrant tub to take a phone call that turned out to be a talking computer that wanted me to buy aluminum siding. Today, I'd give the bath priority.)

Do a little more with your bath than you think you deserve. It's good practice in stretching your ability to love yourself. Does it seem outrageous to you to play Mozart in the bathroom or bathe by candlelight? Do it anyway. There's no better

Playtime

. . . .

Play is as essential for a happy life as are good nutrition, sleep, and exercise. It's an excellent de-stressor that can clear out your thought processes and help you put things into better perspective. Play and creativity are also inextricably linked. When we let our inner child come out to play, original thought often comes, too. Matthew Fox, author of *Creation Spirituality*, wrote that art is "the result of play." Of course, you can lead a loving life without play, but know that it won't be as productive or as enjoyable.

A common complication of addiction is that it can cause people to lose their ability, and even their desire, to play. Since food addiction can start in early childhood, some of us never fully expressed our inherently playful propensities, even at that time in life when play comes most naturally. If we want to play now, we have to learn how to do it.

I was so serious about learning to play and get over my near-terminal seriousness that I actually took a course called "Play for Grown-ups." The teacher, a *professional recreator*, had us hanging from monkey bars and flirting with eternity on a jungle gym from the first night. Soon we worked our way up to hide-and-seek, "Simon says," and stacking ourselves into four-layer human pyramids at the park. It was terrifying, but it was great.

In that class I learned that it isn't only overeaters who can have trouble with play. A lot of people are simply addicted to adulthood. With a strictly adult mindset, play is extraneous, useless, nonproductive, a waste of time. It can even be a little scary.

As science writer K. C. Cole once stated in a *New York Times* article, "Play is out of control. In real play, we try things just to see what happens. In other words, we take risks." In adult-only thinking, risk is justified in business deals, the stock market, and if someone is drowning, but to risk making a fool of oneself at roller-blade class—you've got to be kidding!

So don't start with roller-blades. Start where you're almost comfortable. My play-class teacher did warn against card games, board games, and sports in the beginning since they're taken way too seriously. Beyond that, it's up to you. Here are some suggestions for gently re-entering the world of play:

- *Develop a better opinion of goofing off.* A lot us have trouble with play because we really believe that there's something wrong about not constantly working, worrying, eating, exercising, or being in some other way purposefully occupied.

Playtime (*continued*)

· · · · · · · · · · · · · · ·

- *Rethink the idea of payoffs.* It's true that play does good things for the mind and body, but it interferes with genuine playfulness if you're thinking, "This game of tag with my kid is reducing my work-related anxieties, developing a closer parent/child bond, and firming my quadriceps muscles."

- *Come at play through the back door.* Befriend its cousin, laughter. Get some humor into your life every day. Read the comics. See a really funny movie. When you laugh, you're enjoying yourself without inhibitions. The same thing happens in play.

- *Observe the play experts: children and animals.* After a while, you may even want to join in their games.

- *Cultivate friends who are playful by nature.* They're the ones who seem to take life lightly. When you look for them, you'll find them.

- *Liberate your own playfulness.* If you feel like singing when you walk, sing when you walk. They do it in Rogers and Hammerstein musicals all the time.

- *Take a playful attitude into the rest of your life.* This isn't to say that there aren't times to be serious, but a person who knows how to play realizes that most things aren't nearly as serious as we make them. Because that person doesn't see every incident as infinitely grave, he or she can be most effective in those rare situations that truly are.

place to begin than in the privacy of the bath. (This is also a good place to start appreciating your body. Look at it kindly, touch it with care, and talk to your body. It will respond.)

Also, consider the quality of the water in which you bathe or shower. Your skin is capable of absorbing some chemical contaminants. For this reason, a shower-filter (check out www.showerfilterstore.com) may be an investment in your wellbeing.

To love yourself internally with water, you'll need to obtain the purest drinking water you can. As hard as it is to believe, our bodies are more than half water, and the water we drink, like the food we eat, really does become us. You have no doubt read that it's good to drink lots of water (six to eight eight-ounce glasses a day according to most health experts). We do need a great deal of water for our systems to function properly. If you're eating an abundance of fresh, raw fruits and vegetables, though, these are largely comprised of water. Therefore, you don't have to drink all the water you need since you'll be eating some of it.

The water you drink should not come from the tap without some serious filtering. Agricultural runoff and other pollutants enter the groundwater, which is then treated with chlorine in city water systems. Chlorine kills germs, but it does nothing to mitigate chemical pollutants. It is, as we discussed in the section on swimming, a potent chemical itself.

Seek out a dependable dealer and have water delivered to your home in returnable containers (glass containers if possible; plastic can leach into the water), or look into a home purification unit (reverse-osmosis gets the highest marks). Use this water for preparing all your foods and beverages, for making ice cubes, and for drinking.

And remember the Earth by refilling the bottle you take to work, the gym, and elsewhere from your pure-water source at home. Those little plastic water bottles everybody is carrying (and tossing) these days are causing a huge problem for landfills. Even recycling lags far behind reusing when you're trying to save a planet.

Love Yourself with Sunlight

Sunlight—enough but not too much—is a necessity for plants to grow, for children to grow, and for life to exist on Earth. We've been well warned about the dangers of excessive sun exposure. Particularly at this time in history when the thinning of the ozone layer is causing more radiation from the sun to permeate the Earth's atmosphere, baking your body in the sun or on a tanning bed is both a cosmetic indiscretion and an invitation to potentially fatal skin cancer. Nevertheless, you can also drown in water, exercise to the point of exhaustion, or rest so much that you never get anything done. This doesn't mean that you should never bathe, exercise, or rest. We need sunlight. We simply have to approach it with intelligence and respect.

A fascinating book on the subject is *Sunlight* by Zane R. Kime, M.D. In his book, Dr. Kime cites scientific studies demonstrating the beneficial effects of exposure to sunlight for a variety of medical conditions. Unlike many of his colleagues who tell their patients to avoid the sun as much as possible, Dr. Kime recommends modest but regular sun exposure geared to individual skin type and the climate in which a person lives.

One of Dr. Kime's most fascinating contentions—one he documents from scientific literature—is the sunlight/nutrition connection. He writes: "Unless one has a proper diet, sunlight has an ill effect on the skin. This must be emphasized: Sunbathing is dangerous for those who are on the standard high-fat American diet or do not get an abundance of vegetables, whole grains, and fresh fruits. Those on the standard high-fat diet should stay out of the sun and protect themselves from it, but at the same time they will suffer the consequences of both the high-fat diet and the deficiency of sunlight." Dr. Kime recommends a vegetarian diet of unrefined foods with ample representation from those foods rich in vitamins C and E and beta-carotene, abundant in yellow and leafy green vegetables.

When you and the sun get together, use your head to give the best to your body. Appreciate what sunny weather does for your disposition. When a day is really glorious, don't shut yourself off from it. Have breakfast on the patio or take a walk during your coffee break. Take advantage of every beautiful day. For safety in the sun, remember Dr. Kime's dietary suggestions and stick with natural foods, avoiding animal fats and most extracted oils.

Protect your skin by wearing a barrier sun-block daily on those constantly exposed areas: face, lips, décolleté, hands. A barrier block is one that protects with a physical shield rather than a chemical reaction. Active ingredients are titanium dioxide and/or micronized zinc oxide. (The brand I use is Dr. Hauschka—www.drhauschka.com—found at health food stores and select independent pharmacies.) Add a brimmed hat in summer and gloves when you drive. The rest of your body can handle some direct sun and will appreciate it.

Remember, there's a difference between spending time outdoors on a bright morning or afternoon and lying on a beach at midday. One is safe and healthful, the other foolhardy. When you approach the sun, follow Dr. Doug Graham's "baby rule": you wouldn't put a baby out in the noonday sun, but you wouldn't keep a baby indoors all the time either. Baby yourself.

Love Yourself with Peace of Mind

The body and the emotions are intimately connected and interdependent. Many of the physical practices alluded to in this section—enjoying sunlight, getting enough rest, energizing with exercise—are natural antidepressants. Eating whole, natural foods also fosters emotional wellbeing because the brain is part of the body and is nourished by the same foods that nourish every other part of you.

Just as positive and negative physical actions can positively and negatively affect our emotions, emotions can in turn affect us physically. We've all experienced this mind/body interaction: feeling our faces flush when we're embarrassed, getting sweaty palms or butterflies in the stomach when we're nervous, or salivating at the very thought of sucking a lemon or biting into a sour pickle. Most overeaters have also seen that bouts of compulsive eating can be tied to anger, fear, or some unidentified emotional malaise.

The science of psychoneuroimmunology deals with how the mind affects the body. It presents convincing evidence that love, joy, laughter, gratitude, and hope can prevent and may even help cure disease. The implication is that happiness doesn't just feel good, it does good.

No one could be happy all the time if that meant being elated, giddy, and ecstatic nonstop. No rational person would expect to sustain such an emotional peak. Besides, we couldn't if we wanted to because those extremes come in response to external events—events over which we have little (if any) control. The kind of happiness we can depend on is *contentment*. It's not exciting like elation, giddiness, and ecstasy, but it's only minimally dependent upon outside happenings. We learned earlier that the body seeks to maintain homeostasis (balance). The mind does, too. When your mind is in a state of balance, contentment is commonplace. You can call it serenity, equanimity, emotional poise, or peace of mind. By any name, it's great stuff.

Certainly things can happen in life that could shake the serenity of a saint, but balanced people have a high contentment quotient and they quickly regain a comfortable level of calmness. This occurs in spite of what's going on around them. Besides, it's not usually some major calamity that interferes with our happiness.

"Nobody has ever tripped over Pike's Peak," my friend Mary Beth used to tell me. "It's the little stuff that will get you."

The starting place for dealing with this little stuff (and more serious challenges) is the same place you started at in dealing with your food addiction: surrender. Leave the outcome up to God.

Surrendering the outcome doesn't mean doing nothing to help yourself. Think of your Higher Power as an orchestra conductor and yourself as one of the musicians. The musicians certainly aren't "doing nothing." They're making the beautiful music—but they do it under the direction of a conductor. Like those musicians, we're at our best when we do what we can and refrain from doing what we can't.

Two things we cannot do are change other people and avert natural law. Who would try anything that ridiculous? We would. We have. We've tried to change people by getting thinner (so he or she would be attracted to us), by working harder (so our bosses would like us better), and by being more self-sacrificing (so our children would appreciate us).

We've attempted to get around natural law, too—usually the laws of physiology ("This box of cookies doesn't count because I'm starting a diet tomorrow" may sound familiar), as well as looking for myriad ways to lose weight without giving up the food fix. When we stop trying to change others and circumvent the laws of nature, we can get busy with those actions that are ours to take on our own behalf. These are the actions that give us peace of mind. They include:

Doing all we can to live in accordance with what we believe to be the will of our Higher Power. Peace Pilgrim, a remarkable woman who taught that inner peace was the prerequisite for world peace, was fond of saying, "Live up to the highest light you have, and more light will be given you."

Allowing ourselves to be changed. Many of us have been self-help experts. We've done everything to change ourselves. Allowing ourselves to be changed is something else. The phrase that fits here is, "Let go and let God."

Performing the next task that's ours to do. The Buddhists have a lovely concept called *dharma.* It translates roughly as *duty.* Every person has a dharma, a calling or purpose, distinctly his or her own. We can work ourselves into a frenzy trying to do someone else's dharma, but when we're committed to finding and doing our own, peace comes with it.

Treating ourselves with respect and expecting the same from others. We show self-respect with respectful thoughts about ourselves and respectful actions toward ourselves. Healthy self-respect doesn't allow us to play roles like victim and martyr. We learn to detach emotionally or separate physically from harmful relationships.

Learning to accept or change negative circumstances. Sometimes we need to temporarily accept a not-so-perfect situation, like a job that doesn't use our skills or an apartment with noisy neighbors. In cases like these, we need to stay put until we find another job or can get out of the lease. We up the odds for doing this with equanimity if we give our highest good not just temporary comfort, the priority. In fact, changing and accepting are the only healthy options in any situation. We all know this deep down. That's why "The Serenity Prayer" has such wide appeal: "Grant me the serenity to *accept* the things I cannot change, the courage to *change* the things I can. . . ."

Accepting is rarely easy because we're accustomed to exerting control. Even the phrase "exerting control" makes my jaw tighten and my shoulder muscles tense. It takes a change in vantage point for peace of mind to become natural for us. Most people can't make the shift without some help. The Twelve Step programs are excellent resources for this help because the steps heal emotionally as well as physically and spiritually. Practicing them to recover from a food addiction (or from any addiction) brings about a noteworthy degree of emotional poise and inner peace.

In addition to a support group, professional counseling can be useful. If you had counseling when you were involved in food addiction (whether you were practicing compulsive eating or compulsive dieting), it may have seemed like a waste of money and time. Do consider it again if you feel the need. You're bound to find the experience far more meaningful when you enter it without the impermeable barrier of active addiction between you and the help being offered. Remember that the therapist works for *you*. You have to like this person and feel safe with him or her. One that I respect has printed on her business cards, "Counsel, Insight, Perspective." If that isn't what you're getting for your $150 an hour, see somebody else.

As you grow spiritually and live addiction-free, your overall stress level will decrease. Part of this will reflect a change in your attitude: there simply aren't as many things that drive you crazy anymore. And there will be fewer stress factors in your life simply because things will be in better order. (For example, you'll keep change in the car so you won't have to worry about having coins for parking meters.) If you need additional stress management techniques, try meditation, affirmations, and prayer; vigorous physical activity; massage and other bodywork; relaxation procedures such as yoga (the breathing practices, in particular) or self-hypnosis; play and laughter; sitting with your feelings (refer to the "Sit with Your Feelings" section in Chapter Three); talking out feelings with another person; spending time in nature or with a companion animal; or keeping a journal.

These are wonderful practices, but I'm not a big fan of the term *stress management*. We tend to "manage" everything far too much. I see gentle helpers like meditation and relaxation less as stress managers than as stress *embracers*. The best information I was given for dealing with my daughter's fussiness during her "terrible two's" was to take her into my arms when she was out of control and hold her securely. It was sometimes a tricky maneuver—if you've been around tearful two-year-olds, you know that they can be pretty slippery—but it nearly always worked. Her sobs would melt into whimpers, her muscles would relax, and we'd be able to rock and talk, pet the kitty, and put the crisis behind us.

The techniques listed here can embrace stress in much the same way that one can embrace a troubled child. When I do this for myself, whatever is causing me stress seems to loosen up and let go. When I take the time to use any of the calming techniques available to me, I see that I'm really embracing that childlike part of myself. When that part in any of us is comforted and content, we really don't need much more.

The Love and Power of Compassion

Compassion is one gift of a love-powered life. If we were indeed separate from one another, separate from the Earth, and separate from our spiritual essence, selfishness would be the winning ticket. Compassion—that ability to "feel with" others—

would be expendable; it could even be a detriment. As things really are, each of us only appears to be an independent entity. At a very basic level, we are a part of all humankind and a part of all livingkind. It benefits us to think of others, not because there's some cosmic tally system of rewards and punishments, but because the compassion we share with each other is shared with the whole, ourselves included. For recovering food addicts, compassion is indispensable because it's the opposite of selfishness. Addiction cannot exist without selfishness, just as fire cannot exist without oxygen.

Selfishness manifests itself in many ways. Surprisingly enough, self-effacement, self-denial, and self-hate are among them. These aren't only negative and damaging, they're self-centered. Compassion, on the other hand, extends to those around us as well as to ourselves. It's all-inclusive. Our underlying connectedness makes this so.

In spite of the apparent separateness of everyone and everything, numerous individuals and even entire civilizations have seen a fundamental unity within this diversity. The Native American worldview traditionally celebrated the interconnectedness of all life. Aldous Huxley, the author of dozens of short story collections and essays, called this "The Perennial Philosophy" and wrote a book by that title.

Many people have come to an inner sense of this oneness, having had what we refer to as a spiritual experience, a unique state in which a person is intensely aware of the unity—and some would say the divinity—of all life. We call these people mystics and think of them as different from the rest of us. I see them only as people who have traveled to a place I've never been and come back different.

Not only have visionaries and idealists glimpsed this oneness of all life but many contemporary scientists have as well. From the viewpoint of the new physics, Fritjof Capra, Ph.D., author of *The Tao of Physics*, writes, "Quantum theory forces us to see the universe not as a collection of physical objects but rather as a complicated web of relations between the various parts of a unified whole."

The natural response to this verity is compassion, expressed in a variety of ways. When it becomes a factor in your food choices, as it is in a love-powered diet, get ready for amazing things to happen.

Choosing foods based on your relationship with the Earth and your relationship with others makes compassionate living more than just a food issue. It touches every facet of your life. Compassion is an attitude with actions and resultant consequences. You may take compassionate action in ways that I haven't discovered yet. I may have come upon some areas of compassionate living that are new to you.

We all benefit when we can learn from each other. Consider these ways to incorporate more compassion into your life:

Revise your definition of compassion. It isn't pity. It's not the province of the goody two-shoes and the bleeding heart. The compassionate person has simply developed an aptitude for caring, like the artist develops an aptitude for painting. The only difference is that as human beings we all have an innate talent for compassion.

Enlarge your capacity to nurture. We nurture ourselves and others when we accept that all people and all creatures have needs, that it's all right to have needs, and that doing what we can to meet them can be fulfilling.

Retire as a judge. Stepping down from the bench relieves you of the responsibility of evaluating every person and situation in your life.

Release your expectations. Addictive people often think that they can save the world. We can't. We can do our part and release the rest.

Permit other people to be themselves. Just because you change doesn't mean everyone else wants to. Resist the temptation to help them out too much. Perhaps their opportunities to grow are coming in other ways.

Listen. Without giving advice, parading your wisdom, or trying to fix anything, listen to the other person. Also listen to your body, to nature, and to those subtle inklings from your intuition.

Extend your circle of compassion. "Until he extends the circle of his compassionate embrace to all living things, man will not himself find peace," wrote Dr. Albert Schweitzer, author of *The Spiritual Life.*

Realize that little things count. One phone call can make a person's day. Recycling one aluminum can saves enough energy to run a TV for three hours. Little things add up.

Become a compassionate consumer. We tend to make purchases because a certain product is our regular brand, it catches our eye, or it's on sale this week. Compassion can be as much of an influence as habit, eye appeal, and price. Our buying habits have far-reaching effects. We need to ask questions: "Was this cleaning product cruelly tested on animals in a laboratory? Is this shirt a bargain because it was made using sweatshop labor?" When we shop compassionately, we're also shopping consciously, freeing ourselves from the hypnotic lure of the marketplace.

Treat yourself with compassion. When we ease up on ourselves, we tend to ease up on those around us. We come to expect less perfection from people and circumstances and appreciate the beauty in imperfect people and things.

Reflect from time to time on how your actions affect the whole. This not only shows you where you might do better but also serves as a reminder of the many areas in which you're already doing very well. Seeing the beneficial impact that your life is having makes you feel good about who you are.

Make compassionate living an adventure. Get excited about being a part of what the late theologian Dr. Ernest Wilson was fond of calling "the upward progression of the universe."

Trust that you'll be OK. Inordinate worry about our own welfare impedes our ability to feel and show compassion. The antidote to this self-centered worry is faith. If faith sounds too much like Sunday morning, try the definition from C. Norman Shealy, M.D., Ph.D.: "Faith is believing that the purpose of life is good even if you can't figure it out."

Take the time to reach out. Everyone is busy, but our success doesn't necessarily correspond with how busy we are. Some of the most successful people are the least hurried. They know that there's time for what's important, and sharing compassion is important.

Give your compassion the opportunity to grow. Don't push yourself into actions that seem absurd to you. If, however, you find yourself catching an uninvited insect and releasing it outside instead of reaching for the bug spray, don't think you've lost your mind. You may instead have found your heart.

As you apply more compassion in various areas of your life, remember that compassion is not a form of barter, a way to get Brownie points with God. The fact that we're capable of living compassionately is itself a gift. When my primary avocation was binge eating, I was in awe of the people who seemed so effortlessly able to be available for others. Some were literacy volunteers. Others provided foster homes for stray dogs and cats. Many planted flowers.

It was the ones who planted flowers that fascinated me most. They always seemed to be saying something like, "My begonias are out!" I never knew if they were onto something—I mean, is it really that magnificent to have your begonias in bloom?—or if they merely got a kick out of petty foolishness. It was when they brought cuttings around so everybody else could grow begonias that I got an inkling of what was going on. Planting something in the earth is a true show of compassion. Watering and waiting while a flower blooms in its own time, and then appreciating and sharing its beauty with others is about as sublime a chain of events as this world can offer.

I wanted this in my life, but when I tried to emulate these people, it never worked. It was like trying to stay on a diet. My version of compassionate living was to compulsively care for the rest of the world, ignore my own needs, and end up feeling resentful. Or I'd throw myself into causes and burn out before the first victory because I'd written so many letters, made so many phone calls, and attended so many committee meetings that I was almost too tired to care what happened. It became apparent that freedom from addiction, healthy balance, and the compassion that would make my life count for something wouldn't result from my best efforts at self-improvement. Freedom, balance, and compassion were already within me, as they are in you. In love-powered living they blossom, along with the begonias.

CHAPTER TEN

FOREVER AFTER

In a standard weight-loss book, this would be the chapter on maintenance, "keeping it off." In love-powered living, however, these terms have little relevance. *Maintenance* implies continual, even laborious, upkeep, as in "The house was OK; it was the maintenance that killed us." Besides, *keeping it off* is, if you think about it, a rather bizarre phrase. The implication is that fat reserves already burned for energy are somehow waiting to jump back on you like a friendly pup unless you're vigilant about "keeping it off."

Sure, I know the theory that fat cells, once developed, only shrink but never go away. If you were overweight as a child, the curse of the greedy fat cells is even worse. The scaremongers will tell you that those hungry cells are lying in wait to make you overeat so they can puff up to their previous size and stature. You already know that I have no medical credentials to debunk a medical theory. I can, however, tell you that I was fat from before I could toddle. Despite this, in the twenty-five years that I've been living in love-powered fashion (and not doing it perfectly, by the way), I haven't once been besieged by an army of fat cells trying to get me to eat stuffed pizza. The same holds true for the hundreds of people I've personally known and worked with who have also rebuilt their bodies in love-powered fashion.

Let's do a rethink on this maintenance idea. Your job is not to maintain a weight loss. One stat I found claims that only two percent of people who lose over twenty-five pounds keep from regaining the weight within seven years. Why go with odds like that? Instead have as your job *maintaining your spiritual connection.* Then your Higher Power stays in charge and you stay addiction-free one day at a time. The old odds become meaningless and your "weight maintenance" is on a completely different basis.

Besides, this time there's no weight-loss diet to be followed by a maintenance diet. Reasonable eating is reasonable eating. If you're normally a 130-pound woman and you eat what a 130-pound woman needs, you'll eventually reach 130 pounds, whether you start at 135 or 150 or 300. You don't have to eat any differently when your weight reaches a certain point. There are also no formerly verboten foods to add back when your body is at a size that pleases you. The only foods you've chosen not to eat *now* are the same foods you won't want to eat *ever* because doing so would keep you from showing love to yourself and others. Being at a comfortable body weight isn't going to cause you to love yourself and others less.

But the most important reason that weight maintenance is not really an issue is that weight itself was never really the issue. It was an aftereffect. These are the facts:

- Addictive eating is an illness. It can recur. When conditions invite it (e.g., dismantling your spiritual connection, deciding to run the show) addictive eating will recur, regardless of body size
- Like other addictions, this one has a spiritual solution. It involves surrender to a loving Higher Power, cleaning up your life in general, and helping other sufferers
- Living in this solution on a daily basis will prevent circumstances from developing that are conducive to relapse
- Living in the solution means continuing what works to help you live addiction-free.

Practicing the last three of the Twelve Steps on an ongoing basis is an excellent way to ensure the spiritual growth that crowds out obsession. Those steps involve continued personal inventory, prayer and meditation, sharing with others, and incorporating spiritual principles into every facet of your life. It's wise to make these steps an everyday practice even (and perhaps especially) after you've lost the weight.

The tricky part about going on with recovery when your body is the way you want it is that society upholds the myth that food problems belong to fat people. In this instance, ignore society. It hasn't yet permeated the collective consciousness of humanity that food addiction is a disease of the spirit that has various emotional and physical ramifications. We can focus so intently on what we're eating or how much we're eating that the disease of food addiction can color our lives whether we're overeating or not. This is the food obsession that keeps us from dealing with our feelings and with real life.

Coming to grips with feelings through our spirituality and sharing with others also gets sidetracked if we're mirror-conscious. It's not good to take appearances too seriously. I once read about a movie star who said that he keeps his sanity (and his humility) by never reading his own press releases. Like him, we're better off not extrapolating from our success assumptions that aren't valid—for instance, that this is actually *our* success. We do take positive action and we can be proud of that, but we don't engineer our transformation. That's what our Higher Power does.

To better understand how this works, here is a marble analogy that an overeater with strong recovery once used to explain how she stays on an even keel:

When I was just beginning to come to grips with my food addiction, I got an invisible marble bag with no marbles in it. After a while, I realized that the floor around me was covered with marbles of all sizes and colors. I started looking at them and realized that one was the cigarette marble. I picked it up, looked at it, and thought to myself that since I no longer chose to smoke, I could put that marble in the bag. Then I saw the alcohol marble and since I don't choose to drink today, I put that in the bag. I picked up the sugar marble and also placed that one in the bag, then more foods that I feel better not eating were put away.

I then looked around for character defects that I had been practicing all my life. By this time, I'd become aware of many of them and had let them be removed, so I put the marbles for lying and gossiping and some other things in the bag. It goes on and on. When I'm doing what I need to do and letting God do for me what I can't do for myself, the string is drawn tight on that bag of marbles and I'm enjoying life just as it is, not expecting, not anticipating, just enjoying.

Sometimes I stop doing some of the things that ensure good recovery, like reading literature that would help me, writing down my feelings, going to meetings, sharing my secrets, talking with others, and letting God be in charge of my life. Then some of the marbles start to roll out of the bag. At first I don't even realize it, but once I become aware, I can leave the marbles out to trip over or I can choose to pick them up and go back to what works. It isn't a bad thing that the marbles start to roll out: the trouble comes when I forget where they belong.

The ability to notice when we start to lose our marbles (so to speak) is the key to a lifelong reality of freedom from the food fix. If we could keep perfectly in tune with our Higher Power at all times, we wouldn't have to do anything else. But trying to be perfect (instead of perfectly human) is a thankless task. We can, however, do our best to keep a strong connection with a loving God and keep in our lives healthy routines and spiritual practice.

If you start to see the following danger signs, tighten up your spiritual program, get support from your group or your mentor, or read portions of this book again:

- Wanting to eat alone
- Eating larger quantities than usual at more and more meals
- Eating very quickly, taking big bites
- Biting your nails or chewing your hair, pencils, or lots of gum
- Craving certain foods or wanting some foods over and over
- Finding meals unsatisfying (the same meals that were fine last week)
- Rationalizing overeating with thoughts like "I'll skip breakfast tomorrow" or "I'll exercise more"
- Turning to new compulsions, like sex or spending
- Experiencing a return of old binge behaviors without the binge—such as lethargy, isolation, outbursts of temper, or not keeping clean
- Feeling suddenly that you have to lose more weight

Be aware that although these signs can be indicators of incipient relapse, they aren't in themselves relapses. Seeing them is not terrible. It doesn't mean you have

Art Appreciation

. . . .

Many of the models in the magazines have beautiful bodies. Many of the guys on a sports team have beautiful bodies, too. The nudes in the classic paintings, although not the media ideal of our time, also have beautiful bodies.

You may feel singled out in having no waist or having flabby arms, sagging breasts, big hips, big thighs, a big stomach, wrong proportions, and other perceived flaws. In mercilessly scrutinizing these, it's easy to forget that the models in the fashion magazines are usually airbrushed adolescents and the guys on the team look no better than any twenty-year-old who works out. The nudes in the paintings do have big hips, big thighs, and big stomachs, but they're beautiful anyway because that's art. You're art, too. It's time for a little art appreciation.

You've probably been told that a good exercise is to stand naked in front of a full-length mirror and experience the total impact of every lump, bump, and bulge. No. That's art criticism. You've taken this course every semester and you've passed with flying colors. Now you're enrolled in art appreciation. The concept is different. You're not supposed to judge the art (in this case, your body). You're supposed to understand it, find out what the artist had in mind when creating it, and learn why it's one of the greatest works of art of all time.

Your body is a great work of art because of its rarity, beauty, and value. Here's why:

Rarity. This comes from the fact that your body is one of a kind, unique to you. The unlikelihood of a certain sperm fertilizing a certain egg to result in your conception is, when you think about it, astounding. You're special—physically as well as in every other way.

When viewed in a universal sense, physical life itself is rare. Think of the vastness of space, the mind-boggling infinitude of an expanding universe. There may be life elsewhere, but as far as any of us knows for certain, this is it. That makes life on Earth—your life on Earth in your physical body—an extraordinary occurrence.

Beauty. The beauty of your body is a given. Nature is the most skilled artist there is, and every natural creation is beautiful. You claim your beauty the instant you decide to accept it as your birthright. We only think of ourselves as ugly when we compare the way we look to some arbitrary standard. For most of us, that standard comes from the unreal worlds of fashion and entertainment. It's a standard based on profitability, not true human beauty. It's a standard with no roots in reality and one that's subject to change.

211

Art Appreciation (continued)

. . . .

Accept your beauty. It doesn't matter if you're overweight. At many times in history, plumpness has been considered attractive, and to this day in parts of the Middle East and Africa full-blown obesity is a desirable attribute. I know, you don't live in Renaissance Italy or rural Africa, it's healthier to be slim, and you want to wear nice clothes right off the rack. Of course, you deserve to be healthy and to wear whatever you like, but that doesn't mean you can't love yourself as you are today and appreciate yourself throughout your life-long adventure of love-powered living.

Value. Whether you like your body or not, it's of great value to you and to the people who love and depend upon you. Appreciate it. Even talk to it. Say something like, "Body, you and I have been through a lot. I've got a food addiction, so you've been put through tough times along with me. But I'm surrendering that addiction now and putting it in the hands of a loving Power that can take care of me so I can take care of you. I've said disparaging things about you in the past, but I really do love and appreciate you. We're in this together."

You may feel strange talking to your body as if it were something separate from you, but food addicts are separated from their bodies anyway. Talking can help you come together as a healthy whole. The most important thing you can do to reach that end is to deepen your spiritual life every day.

A recovering overeater/bulimic who tried this explains what happened for her: "I can really look in the mirror and like what I see. I attribute this to my daily meditation and to a Higher Power that listens and tells me that I am not the sculptor of my form. I'm learning to love my body because that's what I walk in. I look at myself and at the hurt child that I was and I thank my body for taking care of me so well."

When you honor the rarity, the beauty, and the value of your body, you find that art appreciation really is a snap course.

...

"blown" anything. In fact, seeing them can be good. These signals are like the abdominal pain that gets you to the hospital before your appendix bursts. They're warning signs that something needs to change so you won't have to re-enter the mire of guilt-ridden eating.

Like the woman with the invisible bag of marbles, we can go back to what works for us. It's smart to do that as soon as we realize that something is amiss. Food addiction is no game, and we cannot afford to play games with it. Even so, we don't have to be perfectionists and we don't have to be rigid. One of the joys of love-powered living is that it *is* enjoyable. Being honest is liberating, prayer and meditation are relaxing and comforting, and taking care of our physical bodies makes us feel good inside and out. When the illness is rampant, none of this is motivation enough, but once recovery has begun, a sort of magnetic attraction toward wellness is established. You'll want to stay with what works.

When you look at recovery as something that's for life, flexibility has to be there. Let's say you know how important morning meditation is to your new way of life. It's a weekday morning, you have to take the cat to the vet or the car to the shop, and you simply haven't scheduled enough time for meditation. Have you failed? Of course not. You can pray in the bus on the way to work, and you can remember your Higher Power in all the activities of the day. This has been called "practicing the presence of God." The phrase was coined by a medieval monk but it's every bit as valuable today. You can be reminded of the wonder of life when you see a tree or a flower or a squirrel. You can feel the warmth of love when you're with your child, your mate, or a good friend. And you can experience a miracle when you eat your lunch and it's enough.

Flexible Food

Your food program has to be flexible, too. This is not license to eat for a fix; it's part of your protection from it. For medical, social, financial, or geographic reasons, you may have to make additional alterations at some point in the way you eat.

For example, I've traveled to some faraway places where both the food and the way in which it's prepared are different from what I'm accustomed to. In China, for instance, they put a small plate before each diner and bring out courses one at a time—you're never sure how many courses there'll be. This was disconcerting for the first day or two because I had to be totally dependent upon my body to tell me when it had had enough to eat, without visual cues from a standard-size plate of food. But getting more in touch with my body's signals was something I needed to learn. When I'm open to learning what I need to, I don't have to worry about food—in China or anywhere else.

Food addiction is serious and it can be frightening, but to worry about food (or anything else) is counterproductive. For this day, God takes care of my food. When I allow God to take care of the rest of my life, I have serenity. There's security in having a basic idea about what I'll eat today, but if that changes—if I end up eating at a restaurant instead of at home, for instance—it's all right. God can come to restaurants, too.

If a food situation is troubling, do what you need to. Pray. Call someone. Even leave the place if you have to. Giving up dieting for a love-powered life, however, takes a lot of the food temptation with it. I can say for myself that I don't want to eat animal products because I care about these sentient beings and I don't want to contribute to their suffering and slaughter. I don't want to eat junk food and saturated fats and a lot of refined sugar because I care about me. I want to eat and live in as loving and responsible a manner as I can because I care about the Earth and about what's being left to my own child, my stepchildren, and everybody else's children besides.

Another recovering food addict explains it this way: "I believe that God is extending pure love and support to me and God wants me to spread it around to those I come in contact with, including animals. For me, this means not eating them. Also, I feel that the way I eat is healthful and therefore nurturing. I'm able to be more nurturing to myself than ever, and how I eat is part of that. I want to be kind to myself and kind to our planet and to God's other living creatures."

In this frame of mind, selecting some foods and bypassing others is no longer resisting temptation. With the help of a loving Higher Power, you get that desire-level healing that we talked about earlier. When you have that, there's very little temptation to resist. And if for any length of time you've been eating exceptionally high-quality food—as in a diet comprised largely of raw and living foods—you'll experience such high-level health and wellbeing that the idea of temptation from inferior food will seem laughable.

My life is better now than I could have imagined in the days of binges and remorse. I don't obsess about food because so many other things are more enticing.

Because I have a history of food addiction, it's essential that I pay attention to my spiritual life daily, but I also want to do that because it enriches my life in countless other ways, such as translating some of the general impulsiveness of my personality into creativity, energy, and enthusiasm.

My eating is not perfect either. There are times that I eat a meal, stand up, and realize that I've had too much. There's nothing I can do about it except give the incident to God and forget it. Other times, I eat some food that I know I don't need. I just want it. As long as I can eat it, enjoy it, and accept myself, I'm OK. If I started to develop guilt feelings or if I wanted to continue eating, I'd need to get help—a prayer, a phone call, or an honest talk with another person about ways I may have been deluding myself.

The same system works in other aspects of life. If something is making me uncomfortable, I need to look at it and talk about it. Food addiction doesn't mature in a vacuum, nor does it exist by itself. One of its functions was to protect us from feelings we couldn't handle. Once the food addiction is out of the way, the feelings surface. This is normal; it's to be expected. That's why many people in recovery seek professional counseling. It doesn't mean that their recovery isn't working; it means it's proceeding right on schedule. Until I understood this, I thought that having to deal with old issues negated the growth that I'd made. Instead, I see now, I had to grow to a certain point to be able to look at those issues.

A Spiritual Warranty

Something that all recovering food addicts (and everyone else who loses weight) have to look at is body image. How thin is thin enough? You can get some arbitrary weight from a chart or a memory ("I was 115 pounds on prom night . . .") but I firmly believe that your body has the wisdom to settle at the weight necessary for its optimal functioning. If you exercise regularly, your body will be less fat than it would be at the same weight if you were sedentary. In any case, you'll reach and stay at the size that's right for you by living according to the principles outlined in this book. When you change your diet, not with a specific goal weight in mind but because your life and your world will be better when you do, your body will take it from there.

Forever After

- Never forget that food addiction is a disease. It can reactivate if you cease to nurture its spiritual solution.

- Be honest in all areas of your life, especially about your food and your thoughts about food.

- Stay with your support group, both for what it gives you and for what you bring to it. There and elsewhere, cultivate friendships with positive, accepting people.

- Keep up your spiritual practices, especially the last three of the Twelve Steps, which deal with continued personal inventory, prayer and meditation, sharing recovery, and practicing these principles in all your affairs.

- Cherish your body. It's beautiful. If you can't accept your body as it is, get help from people who have accepted theirs.

- Look out for the signs that your spiritual life may need your attention and make the necessary changes.

- Give your continued health as a whole person a high priority. This includes your physical health, your emotional wellbeing, your relationships, your work, and your finances, as well as your happiness, creativity, and fulfillment.

- Keep your eating flexible and livable. Replace punitive diets with healthful, life-affirming eating habits. Avoid animal foods to the degree that you're willing: remembering that "meat's no treat for those we eat" helps keep your conviction stronger than more selfish motivations. Eat lots of fresh fruits and vegetables, and get into juicing for an infusion of life force every day. Instead of treating yourself with inferior foods, treat yourself well with the foods you eat.

- Exercise regularly in ways that add to the overall quality of your life.

- Express gratitude to God, to life, and to people. Every addict in recovery is a visible miracle. It's easy to get involved with living and forget that. By all means be involved with living, but at least once a day, take the time to count your blessings and be grateful.

This may be the most difficult area of all in which to trust your Higher Power. I can remember hearing a talk by someone I greatly admired about trusting in the will of a loving Higher Power. I believed that God was loving, and I'd long discarded the concept that tragedy and punishment were the ways that God's will manifested itself in my life. I just thought that God couldn't possibly understand about my body. I felt then that I had to be really slender and have those muscles that show—not big ones, just the kind that are apparent because they're taut and aren't competing with fat for visual attention. I also had a goal weight in mind that was as unchangeable as my date of birth or my Social Security number.

Well, I got to my goal weight on a pre-recovery diet. Then I went below my goal weight in pre-recovery insanity. Then I went well above it on a pre-recovery, extended binge. Finally, I gave up the fight. In recovery my body found a weight at which it's comfortable. It's slightly more than my old goal weight and a lot less than what I weighed when I insisted that the number I'd chosen on the scale was the only one I'd accept. I have no ironclad guarantee that I will never gain weight, but my body (and anything else that concerns me) is under a sort of spiritual warranty. The manufacturer takes care of it. The warranty is only invalid if I'm turning to food instead of turning to Spirit. Today's freedom, today's spirituality, and today's contentment are all that any of us gets. As we live in the way that makes these available to us, we have every right to trust that they will be with us forever after. The trust builds on itself.

As another recovering person said: "The more I'm able to trust God and reach out to both God and other people for comfort and healing, the less need I have to eat when I am not hungry. The paradox is this: I am afraid to trust, but the more I trust and put my life in God's hands, the smoother things go. Then it becomes easier to keep on trusting."

That's the trust that allows the power of love into our lives, the love that overcomes addiction and other assorted miseries. I have a sneaking suspicion, however, that just as we need to trust God, there may be ways in which God is trusting us. There are statues and stories, gardens and quilts, and friendships and families that might never exist if we don't create them. There are people and animals and forests and rivers asking for our love and care. It could be that as we trust in our Higher Power to keep us free from obsession one day after another, our Higher Power is trusting in us to form the friendships and plant the gardens.

It's a collective effort, an effort that doesn't leave much time for agonizing over what to have for dinner or what you think of your thighs. Your dinner will be delicious, and your thighs will be just fine. The things you have to attend to are simply more important, more appealing, and more fulfilling. Not only will your meals be comprised of love-powered foods, your days will be filled with love-powered activities. With this combination, you'll like living in your body, and you'll love living your life.

THE TWELVE STEPS

To follow are the Twelve Steps as they come from their source, Alcoholics Anonymous. The word "alcohol" in Step One and the word "alcoholics" in Step Twelve can be changed to make the steps read appropriately for dealing with your food problem.

1. We admitted we were powerless over alcohol—that our lives had become unmanageable.
2. Came to believe that a Power greater than ourselves could restore us to sanity.
3. Made a decision to turn our will and our lives over to the care of God as we understood Him.
4. Made a searching and fearless moral inventory of ourselves.
5. Admitted to God, to ourselves, and to another human being the exact nature of our wrongs.
6. Were entirely ready to have God remove all these defects of character.
7. Humbly asked Him to remove our shortcomings.
8. Made a list of all persons we had harmed and became willing to make amends to them all.
9. Made direct amends to such people wherever possible, except when to do so would injure them or others.

10. Continued to take personal inventory and when we were wrong, promptly admitted it.

11. Sought through prayer and meditation to improve our conscious contact with God as we understood Him, praying only for knowledge of His will for us and the power to carry that out.

12. Having had a spiritual awakening as the result of these steps, we tried to carry this message to alcoholics and to practice these principles in all our affairs.

NUTSHELL NUTRITION

If you're a food addict, you've probably read quite a bit about nutrition. (As a kid, I memorized nutrient charts while my friends read comic books.) Should you need an additional reference, this appendix is quick and to the point: plant-based nutrition in a peapod. We'll start with the big guys or macronutrients: carbohydrates, protein, and fats.

Carbohydrates

Unrefined carbohydrate foods are our foremost energy source and also the storehouses of other vital nutrients. Carbohydrates come as either sugar or starch. Sugars are simple and can be utilized by the body almost immediately. Starches are broken down into sugars during the digestive process. Natural sugars are deliciously packed in fruit, with the highest concentration found in dried fruit. Starch is found in grains, vegetables, and legumes.

Refinement is good for social climbing but bad for carbohydrate nutrition. White sugar is the ultimate in this kind of refinement, so eliminate (or at least drastically cut down on) soft drinks and conventional baked goods. Use sweeteners such as dates, fruit concentrates, maple syrup, and agave nectar (a light, honey-like sweetener that comes from—no kidding—cactus). Remember, however, that all sweetness comes from sugar and even sweeteners from Mother Nature's kitchen can be overdone. One exception is stevia, a calorie-free herb that can be substituted for artificial sweeteners.

Also, read labels. Corn syrup, brown sugar, raw sugar, fructose, dextrose, sucrose, and lactose are all forms of sugar, so beware of any packaged food product with a concentration of one or more of these. (Ingredients are listed on the label in order of the amount contained in the product. Some manufacturers are clever, though, and may use two or three types of sugar so no single one has to be listed as the first or second ingredient.)

Highly processed grains—like white flour, white rice, and degerminated cornmeal—have also been robbed of nutrients. In "enriched" foods, some nutrients are replaced, but enrichment is like having the person who steals your car give you bus fare. Stick with the whole grains and simple cereals, but beware of the old hippie favorite, granola—it's usually high in fat and terribly sweet. Also note that even refined carbohydrates are generally superior to fatty foods. You'd be better off with tofu and broccoli over white rice than with sweet-and-sour pork, or with white-flour pasta and marinara sauce than with veal parmigiana. (Of course, the pig and calf in question have a major stake in your choice as well.)

Protein

Protein is necessary for, among other things, growth, tissue repair, and combating infection. The Daily Value in the United States is fifty grams—well above the World Health Organization's recommendation of thirty-nine grams a day for males and twenty-nine for females. But meeting either standard on a varied, natural, vegetarian diet isn't difficult. It may actually be good to avoid going over the Daily Value very often since calcium depletion and kidney damage are among the problems that have been linked with excess protein consumption.

Amino acids are the units that make up protein. Eight of them, called the essential amino acids, must be supplied by the diet. It was formerly believed that only animal foods provided complete protein (or all the essential amino acids) and that the only way vegetable foods could be made sufficient was to combine different foods (generally grains and legumes) at the same meal to create an amino-acid profile that looked like that of meat. This is not necessary. Simply eat a variety of foods throughout the day and in your diet overall.

Although there are many plant foods that are concentrated proteins, such as peanuts, dried beans and peas, quinoa, hemp seeds, and soy products such as tofu, these do not need to be emphasized. In fact, a cup of beans a day is plenty. And because all natural foods contain some protein, eating a variety of these ensures that you'll get ample protein even on the days you leave beans off the menu.

Fats

Fats provide warmth and a concentrated energy source as well as essential linoleic and linolenic fatty acids. Saturated fats, which aren't necessary for essential fatty acids, are found primarily in animal foods, like butter, cheese, and meat, and in a few plant products, primarily coconut, chocolate, and palm oil. Unsaturated fats are abundant in vegetable oils, nuts, seeds, and avocado.

Although not as damaging as saturated fats and the artificial trans fats that result from hydrogenating oils, excess fat from any source has been linked with high cholesterol levels and increased risk of heart disease, and it may be a factor in the development of certain cancers. The safest course to take is to keep total fat intake modest—no more than twenty percent of calories. The most efficient way to do this is to eliminate most commercial baked goods, fried foods, and animal products, and to be frugal in the use of higher-fat plant foods such as peanut butter and oil-based salad dressings. Using some olive oil is acceptable for most people, but measure it by the spoonful. It's a quality fat but it's still all fat, so don't overdo.

The fats that appear to protect against heart disease (and possibly other conditions that arise from tissue inflammation, such as arthritis) are the omega-3 fatty acids: ALA, EPA, and KHAS. The first is found primarily in plants, the other two in marine sources—fish oil or a supplement derived from algae (where the fish get their omega-3s in the first place). Brands of non-animal omega-3 supplements include Peva, Water of Life, and Health from the Sun.

Note: Despite their omega-3 content, avoiding fish and fish oil is wise due to their contamination with toxins such as mercury, DDT, PCBs, dioxins, lead, and other chem-

icals. This is especially true of predatory species like tuna and swordfish. According to the EPA, women who ate fish more than twice a week were shown to have seven times the mercury in their blood as women who didn't consume fish. In addition, fish are living, feeling creatures. I often hear someone say, "I'm a vegetarian—I just eat fish." A fish is not a vegetable.

Fiber

Fiber (or roughage) isn't really a nutrient, but this indigestible part of plants is important in digestion and elimination. A natural foods diet of vegetables, fruits, whole grains, and legumes is by definition a high-fiber diet, even without supplementary fibers such as wheat bran for bowel regularity or oat bran to lower cholesterol. (Besides, this is a zero-cholesterol diet, which, for most people, should eliminate the need for an extraneous cholesterol-lowering agent.) Meat and most other animal products are virtually fiber-free. Fiber is also lost in processing, so try to choose whole fruits instead of fruit juice and whole-grain bread instead of white, and leave the skins on your potatoes.

The Micronutrients

When it comes to vitamins and minerals, small is mighty. They don't take up much space in your body, but they're important. A natural foods diet is full of vitamins and minerals. And when you consider that nutrition is still a young science with more vital food components yet to be isolated, it's important to choose natural foods that haven't lost their best parts to the mill or the cannery.

Minerals

Minerals are body-building elements that also aid in digestion and temperature regulation. Among the major ones are:

Calcium. Bone and tooth formation, blood clotting, muscle contraction, and nerve transmission require calcium. Because a high protein intake has been shown to deplete the body's calcium stores, people with an adequate but modest protein intake (provided in a plant-based diet) are believed to require less calcium than meat-eaters do. The Daily Value for calcium is a thousand milligrams; the World Health Organization's recommendation, however, is only 500 milligrams per day. Foods rich in calcium include green leafy vegetables (collards and kale top the list), sea vegetables (kelp, dulse, nori), nuts such almonds and hazelnuts, legumes such as chickpeas and pinto beans, calcium-cultured tofu, calcium-fortified orange juice, and calcium-fortified soy and rice milk.

Iodine. A tiny but essential amount (100 to 300 micrograms) is needed for energy production and proper functioning of the thyroid gland. It's added to iodized salt but is also abundant in sea vegetables and in vegetables grown in coastal areas with significant levels of iodine in the soil.

Iron. Needed by the blood for its oxygen supply, this mineral also aids in disease resistance and red blood cell formation. Iron is found in leafy greens (collards, kale, broccoli), legumes (chickpeas, lentils, lima beans), and other foods including whole grains and fruits—dried fruits in particular. Consuming food rich in vitamin C along with iron-rich food increases iron absorption by the body. Premenopausal women, the population group most likely to become anemic, need ten milligrams a day.

Magnesium. Required for the body's acid-alkaline balance and for blood sugar metabolism, magnesium is part of the nutrient package of peanuts, almonds, legumes such as soybeans and lima beans, millet, wheat, and rye. The Daily Value is 400 milligrams.

Phosphorus. Though used in a variety of body processes including energy production, phosphorus is mainly calcium's right-hand mineral, important in bone and tooth development. Phosphorus is widely available in foods, and meeting the thousand-milligram Daily Value for adults is not a problem. Rich sources include whole grains, legumes, peanuts, and peanut butter.

Potassium. Potassium is necessary for proper functioning of the heart and other muscles and for nerves. You can find it in sea vegetables, soybeans and lima beans, dried apricots, sunflower seeds, and prunes.

Selenium. A trace mineral with antioxidant properties, selenium is a component of whole grains, broccoli, nutritional yeast, and onions.

Sodium. Although sodium is lost in sweat, urine, and feces, it's replaced by foods and most people get too much. Table salt is the recognized source of sodium, but milk and its products, meats, canned vegetables, baked goods, and snack foods up the average intake considerably. Adequate sodium is provided by fresh vegetables. Use salt and soy sauce with a light hand.

Zinc. Needed for proper growth, reproduction, immune function, and wound healing, zinc is in oatmeal, peanuts, peas, dried beans, pumpkin seeds, and even popcorn. There's conjecture that phytates in whole grain may inhibit zinc absorption, but this has not been evidenced clinically.

Vitamins

Vitamins are vital to normal metabolism. They are either fat-soluble (vitamins A, D, and E) or water-soluble (vitamins B and C); the latter are more easily lost through careless preparation. Boiling murders vitamins. Make steaming, baking, and stir-frying your cooking methods of choice, and turn any leftover cooking water into soup stock. Better yet, eat raw vegetables whenever possible. If you bypass pale iceberg lettuce for leaf or romaine or nutrient-dense mesclun greens, your salad will be like a multivitamin with dressing.

Vitamin A. For healthy skin, eyes, and respiratory tract, think yellow and dark green—as in sweet potatoes, carrots, cantaloupe, dried apricots, kale, collards, and spinach. The Daily Value for vitamin A is 5,000 international units (IUs).

Vitamin B complex. Needed for digestion, protein breakdown, and nervous system functioning, the Bs aren't called complex for nothing: they're a conglomerate of vitamins. Nutritional yeast (a fortified and tastier form of brewer's yeast) is the classic vitamin B health food, but members of the B family also congregate in whole grains, wheat germ, and peanuts.

Following is a B-by-B breakdown, including some of the richest sources of each.

- B1 (thiamine) contributes to a good appetite and carbohydrate metabolism. Rich sources are brown rice, sunflower seeds, soybeans, and other legumes.
- B2 (riboflavin) contributes to antibody and red blood cell formation, cell res-

piration, and metabolism of all food elements. Good sources are almonds, whole-wheat bread, wild rice, leafy greens, and legumes.

- B4 (niacin) is needed for cell metabolism and respiration as well as carbohydrate absorption. The niacin deficiency disease, pellagra, was common prior to the enrichment of refined grains. Good sources are brown rice, wild rice, peanuts, millet, and collards.
- B6 (pyridoxine) contributes to antibody formation and hydrochloric acid production. Good sources are peppers, leafy greens, cauliflower, citrus fruits, and potatoes.
- B12 (cobalamin) is required by the nervous system and by the blood in minuscule but essential amounts. Since it's produced by microorganisms, most people can probably get all they need from the microbes that live in their mouths and intestines. Because B12 doesn't reliably occur in vegetable foods, however, the wise course for a total vegetarian is to regularly take a supplementary B12 tablet to meet the Daily Value of six micrograms or to regularly use foods fortified with cobalamin.

Vitamin C. Involved in collagen production, digestion, healing, and infection resistance, vitamin C gets to the table in citrus fruits, cantaloupe, strawberries, bell peppers, cabbage-family vegetables, and potatoes. The Daily Value for adults is sixty milligrams per day, although a substantial body of research indicates that a higher intake is optimal.

Vitamin D. The sunshine vitamin is essential for teeth and bones, so it's especially critical for children and pregnant women. Vitamin D is also needed for calcium metabolism and heart action. Although dairy products and margarine are fortified with it, nature intended for us to get vitamin D from a unique chemical reaction of sunlight on our skin.

Vitamin D is stored in our tissues to make up for those times of the year when the sun isn't strong enough to do its part in vitamin D synthesis. Even so, dark-skinned people and anyone living in a northern latitude (as far vitamin D goes, "northern" is the upper third of the U.S.) are hard-pressed to get enough sunlight for this process. In addition, many of us in every location are doing such a good job of protecting our skin from the aging and potentially carcinogenic downside of sun exposure that we're sacrificing vitamin D in the process. Therefore, a supplement of 400 IUs daily, at least in the fall and winter, is strongly recommended.

Vitamin E. Vitamin E is an antioxidant that regulates destructive oxidizing of cell membranes and vitamin A. Rich sources include whole grains, wheat germ, sweet potatoes, leafy greens, and navy beans. The Daily Value for adults is thirty IUs. Vitamin E was once touted as a virtual panacea for heart disease and although the more enthusiastic claims have been widely discounted, many cardiologists still recommend modest supplementation of 200 IUs daily.

RECOMMENDED READING

Recovery from Addiction, Overeating, Overweight

Anonymous. *Alcoholics Anonymous: The Story of How Many Thousands of Men and Women Have Recovered from Alcoholism.* New York: Alcoholics Anonymous World Service, 4th edition, 2001. This is the basic text of Alcoholics Anonymous and the foundation for all the Twelve Step programs. The first section is a veritable recipe for recovery from addiction; the remainder of the book contains inspiring stories of recovered alcoholics.

___. *For Today.* Rio Rancho, N.M.: Overeaters Anonymous, 1982. A lovely little volume of daily meditations specifically for overeaters.

___. *The Twelve Steps and Twelve Traditions.* New York: Alcoholics Anonymous World Service, 2002. A detailed exploration of how alcoholics in AA recover and how the fellowship functions, written by one of the co-founders of Alcoholics Anonymous and originally published in 1952.

___. *The Twelve Steps and Twelve Traditions of Overeaters Anonymous.* Rio Rancho, N.M.: Overeaters Anonymous, 1993. Details the spiritual program of recovery specifically for overeaters. Contains keen insights into compulsive eating as an addiction and presents the steps in a way that's immediately applicable to people who have problems with food.

Burns, John, and other recovered alcoholics. *The Answer to Addiction: The Path to Recovery from Alcohol, Drug, Food, and Sexual Dependencies.* New York: Crossroad Publishing Company, 1990. A profound, no-holds-barred explanation of addiction and its answer using the Twelve Steps.

Crister, Greg. *Fat Land: How Americans Became the Fattest People in the World.* New York: Mariner Books (Houghton Mifflin), 2004. A journalist's exposé of why nearly sixty percent of Americans are overweight. Covers the food we eat, the exercise we're not getting, the role of high fructose corn syrup, and how agribusiness has unwittingly altered the American diet.

Greenberg, Rena. *The Right Weigh: Six Steps to Permanent Weight Loss Used by More than 100,000 People.* Carlsbad, Calif.: Hay House, 2005. The author is a certified hypnotherapist and her program includes knowing your vision, turning to your Source for help, accepting yourself as you are, and reprogramming your subconscious mind.

Hollis, Judi. *Fat is a Family Affair: A Guide for People with Eating Disorders and Those Who Love Them.* Center City, MN: Hazelden Publishing, 1996. A book that has helped food addicts for 29 years.

L., Elizabeth. *Twelve Steps for Overeaters: An Interpretation of the Twelve Steps of Overeaters Anonymous.* Center City, Minn.: Hazelden, 1993. An exploration of the steps to a spiritual experience, explaining with compassion and understanding how chronic overeaters must bring their entire lives, physical and spiritual, into balance.

Moran, Victoria. *Fit from Within: 101 Simple Ways to Change Your Body and Your Life . . . Starting Today and Lasting Forever.* New York: Contemporary Books (McGraw-Hill), 2003. Short, prescriptive essays for overcoming overeating, accepting yourself, and living in the solution.

Roth, Geneen. *Breaking Free from Emotional Eating.* New York: Plume (Penguin), 2003. The beloved author of *Feeding the Hungry Heart* and *When Food Is Love* offers simple techniques and practical advice on eating without distraction, kicking the scale habit, withstanding family and social pressures, and more.

Spirituality, Self-Help, Inspiration

Beak, Sera. *The Red Book: A Deliciously Unorthodox Approach to Igniting Your Divine Spark.* San Francisco: Jossey-Bass (Wiley), 2006. Ostensibly a spirituality book geared to women in their twenties, this groundbreaking work by a young, Harvard-trained theologian speaks to anyone who sees the life of the spirit as an enticing adventure.

Friends of Peace Pilgrim. *Peace Pilgrim: Her Life and Work in Her Own Words.* Santa Fe: Ocean Tree Books, 1992. A compilation of the wisdom of this modern mystic who walked across America for nearly three decades carrying the message: "This is the way to peace—Overcome evil with good, and falsehood with truth, and hatred with love."

Hay, Louise. *You Can Heal Your Life.* Carlsbad, Calif.: Hay House, 1999. Affirmations, positive thinking, seeing yourself as God sees you—a great help on the spiritual path and to support physical and emotional healing.

Huxley, Aldous. *The Perennial Philosophy.* New York: Perennial Classics (Harper-Collins), 2004, originally published by Harper and Brothers, 1945. Huxley's exhaustive but eminently readable treatise on the mystical underpinnings of the world's spiritual teachings.

Moran, Victoria. *Creating a Charmed Life: Simple, Spiritual Secrets Every Busy Woman Should Know.* San Francisco: HarperSanFrancisco, 1999. Little classic in short-essay format for living the life you want.

_____. *Fat, Broke & Lonely No More: Your Personal Solution to Overeating, Overspending, and Looking for Love in All the Wrong Places.* San Francisco: HarperOne, 2007. Guide to overcoming the inner emptiness that can lead to problems with food, money, and relationships.

Powers, Thomas. *Invitation to a Great Experiment: Exploring the Possibility that God Can Be Known.* New York: Crossroad Publishing, 1990. The frontispiece of this book is a photo of an alarm clock, supporting the claim that if you want to know God you start by getting up an hour earlier each day for study, prayer/meditation, and physical exercise.

Shinn, Florence Scovel. *The Florence Scovel Shinn Reader: The Game of Life; Your Word Is Your Wand; The Power of the Spoken Word; The Secret Door to Success.* Camarillo, Calif.: DeVorss Publications, 2007. Compilation of the four books of this twentieth-century metaphysical teacher who had "the secret" a long time ago.

Nutrition, Health, Weight Loss

Barnard, Neal D., M.D. *Breaking the Food Seduction: The Hidden Reason Behind Food Cravings—and 7 Steps to End Them Naturally.* New York: St. Martin's Press, 2003. Reveals how simple dietary and lifestyle changes can break the stubborn cycle of cravings for sweets and high-fat foods. With recipes by Joanne Stepaniak.

_____. *Dr. Neal Barnard's Program for Reversing Diabetes: The Scientifically Proven System for Reversing Diabetes without Drugs.* In a series of studies, Dr. Barnard found it possible to repair insulin function and reverse Type II diabetes through a diet of vegetables, fruits, whole grains, and legumes. Recipes from Bryanna Clark Grogan.

Campbell, T. Colin, Ph.D., and Thomas M. Campbell II. *The China Study: Startling Implications for Diet, Weight-Loss and Long-Term Health.* Dallas: BenBella Books, 2006. Results from the largest nutritional study ever conducted show that a plant-based, whole-foods diet can dramatically reduce the risk of cancer, heart disease, diabetes, and obesity.

Chopra, Deepak, M.D. *Perfect Health: The Complete Mind/Body Guide.* New York: Three Rivers Press, 2000. A life-affirming guide to good health based on the ancient Indian healing system of Ayurveda; includes a section on freedom from addictions.

Dupont, Caroline Marie. *Enlightened Eating: Nourishment for Body and Soul.* Burnaby, B.C., Canada: Alive Books, 2007. Holistic nutritionist offers natural ways to consume a more plant-based diet, with healthy recipes and inspiration.

Esselstyn, Caldwell B., M.D. *Prevent and Reverse Heart Disease: The Revolutionary, Scientifically Proven, Nutrition-Based Cure.* New York: The Penguin Group, 2007. How a low-fat, plant-based diet was shown through decades-long research at the Cleveland Clinic to reverse cardiovascular disease; how to implement the program for yourself; and non-intimidating recipes.

Freedman, Rory, and Kim Barnouin, *Skinny Bitch: A No-nonsense Tough-love Guide for Savvy Girls Who Want to Stop Eating Crap and Start Looking Fabulous.* Philadelphia: Running Press, 2005. A young, hip, in-your-face guide to eating plant-based foods for health, beauty, and pizzazz.

Freston, Kathy. *Quantum Wellness: The Practical and Spiritual Guide to Health and Happiness.* New York: Weinstein Books, 2008. Focused, small steps to health and contentment including conscious eating (working toward a vegan diet for the good of all), meditation, visualization, fun, exercise, self-work, spiritual practice, and service.

Fuhrman, Joel, M.D. *Eat to Live: The Revolutionary Plan for Fast and Sustained Weight Loss.* Boston: Little, Brown & Co., 2003. Based on Fuhrman's brilliant "nutrient density" concept, this book shows that when the ratio of nutrients to calories is high, fat is lost and health triumphs.

Goldbeck, Nikki, and David Goldbeck. *Healthy Highways: The Travelers' Guide to Healthy Eating.* Woodstock, N.Y.: Ceres Press, 2004. Lists 1,900 healthy eateries and natural food stores throughout the U.S., along with state maps and local directions.

Havala, Suzanne, M.S., R.D. *Being Vegetarian for Dummies.* New York: Hungry Minds, Inc., 2001. The acclaimed dietitian Suzanne Havala Hobbs gets you started, provides nutritional info, helps you deal with social concerns, and makes it easy to go veg in the real world.

McDougall, John, M.D. *The McDougall Program for Maximum Weight Loss.* New York: Plume (Penguin), 1995. A guide to adopting a low-fat, health-supporting diet for lasting weight loss. With recipes by Mary McDougall.

Oski, Frank A., M.D. *Don't Drink Your Milk! New Frightening Medical Facts about the World's Most Overrated Nutrient.* Brushton, N.Y.: Teach Services, 1992. The director of the Department of Pediatrics at Johns Hopkins University School of Medicine offers a strong case for wiping off your milk mustache.

Robbins, John. *The Food Revolution: How Your Diet Can Help Save Your Own Life and Our World.* Berkeley: Conari Press, 2001. Describes the health effects of what we eat, genetically modified food, how to extend life, increase vitality, and build a more compassionate and sustainable world. (Statistics from this exhaustively researched book are distilled in the booklet *Our Food Our Future: Making a Difference with Every Bite* from EarthSave International: www.earth-save.org.)

Ethics, Humanity, Sustainability

Baur, Gene. *Farm Sanctuary: Changing Hearts and Minds About Animals and Food.* New York: Touchstone Books (Simon & Schuster). Tells the story of the first sanctuary for farm animals, explains current agricultural methods, and encourages looking at farm animals as beings in their own right (a process aided by the fascinating individuals rescued by Farm Sanctuary and introduced, with photos, in the book).

Lyman, Howard. *Mad Cowboy: Plain Truth from the Cattle Rancher Who Won't Eat Meat.* New York: Touchstone (Simon & Schuster), 2001. Fourth generation Montana rancher blasts through the propaganda of the meat and dairy interests.

Masson, Jeffrey Moussaieff. *The Pig Who Sang to the Moon: The Emotional World of Farm Animals.* New York: Ballantine Books (Random House), 2004. Masson weaves history, literature, anecdotes, scientific studies, and five years of his own experiences observing pigs, cows, sheep, goats, and chickens to shatter the cruel myth that the animals we eat are without feelings.

Rice, Pamela. *101 Reasons Why I'm a Vegetarian.* New York: Lantern Books, 2005. A compelling volume covering every incentive from cholesterol to mad cow; hormones in meat and milk to heart failure, stroke, and bypass; animal abuse to laborers exploited.

Robbins, John. *Diet for a New America.* Tiburon, Calif.: H. J. Kramer, Inc., in conjunction with New World Library, Novato, Calif., 1998. A modern classic that explores the positive impact of a totally vegetarian diet on other animals, our own health, and the health of the planet.

Tuttle, Will, Ph.D. *The World Peace Diet: Eating for Spiritual Health and Social Harmony.* New York: Lantern Books, 2005. An enlightened look at food choices and how changing them could help us move toward a freer and happier world.

Cookbooks

*Note: For some compulsive eaters in the early stages of recovery, cookbooks are binge trig-
gers. If this is the case for you, stick with simple foods, easily prepared, and save the
cookbooks for later. In time, you'll find that your life can accommodate every good
thing—cookbooks, too.*

Atlas, Nava. *Vegan Express.* New York: Broadway Books, 2008. Quick, delicious,
healthy recipes with lots of international dishes.

Feral, Priscilla, Lee Hall, and Friends of Animals, Inc. *Dining with Friends: The Art
of North American Vegan Cuisine.* Darien, Conn.: Friends of Animals, 2005. A
beautiful collection of simple but elegant recipes for every occasion.

Freedman, Rory, and Kim Barnouin. *Skinny Bitch in the Kitch: Kick-Ass Recipes for
Hungry Girls Who Want to Stop Cooking Crap (and Start Looking Hot!).* Philadelphia: Running Press, 2007. *New York Times* bestseller from the *Skinny Bitch*
gals, with sections including "Grown-Up Appetizers," "Sassy Soups and Stews,"
and "Happy Endings" (desserts).

McCarthy, Brian P. *The Lantern Vegan Family Cookbook.* New York: Lantern Books,
2005. Chef McCarthy features family-pleasing vegan versions of traditional
recipes (over 400 in all) including pizza, quiche, French toast, and eggnog.

Moskowitz, Isa Chandra, and Terry Hope Romero. *Veganomicon: The Ultimate
Vegan Cookbook.* New York: Marlowe & Co. (Avalon Publishing Group), 2007.
Two top vegan chefs present 250 delicious recipes and include soy-free, gluten-
free, and low-fat choices.

People for the Ethical Treatment of Animals, including recipes from Bryanna Clark
Grogan and Louise Hagler. *Cooking with PETA: Great Recipes for a Compassionate Kitchen.* Summertown, Tenn.: The Book Publishing Company, 1997. Favorite vegan dishes from PETA staffers. Yummies include "Tasty Toona Salad,"
"Beefless Stew," and "Tofu Not-a-Turkey."

Pierson, Joy, Bart Potenza, and Barbara Scott Goodman. *The Candle Café Cookbook:
More than 150 Enlightened Recipes from New York's Renowned Vegetarian Restaurant.* New York: Clarkson Potter, 2003. Candle Café has been a haunt for
healthy New Yorkers since Gloria Swanson went there for juice in the forties and

fifties. In its present incarnation, this happening East Side eatery and its up-scale sibling, Candle 79, meld whole ingredients and gourmet sensibilities. The cookbook follows suit.

Stepaniak, Joanne. *The Uncheese Cookbook.* Summertown, Tenn.: The Book Publishing Company, 1994. Dairy-free cheese substitutes and classic "uncheese" dishes.

Tucker, Eric, John Westerdahl, Sascha Weiss. *The Millennium Cookbook: Extraordinary Vegetarian Cuisine.* Berkeley: Ten Speed Press, 1998. The subtitle says it all; the cuisine really is extraordinary, coming as it does from San Francisco's august Millennium Restaurant. The recipes take some doing and the results are more than worth it.

Raw Foods

Butler, Lillian R., and Eddie D. Robinson. *Health Journey: Your Personal Road Map for Vibrant Living and Youthful Aging.* New York: Labor of Love Productions, LLC, 2008. Owners of the popular Harlem eatery Raw Soul (www.rawsoul.com) have created this compact and jam-packed guide to natural living, vegan/whole-foods nutrition, and raw foods. Topics include hydration, food combining, juice fasting, exercise, making changes last, and a restaurant-tested recipe section.

Cohen, Alissa. *Living on Live Food.* Kittery, Me.: Cohen Publishing Co., 2004. Exquisite, glossy 550-page tome in two parts. The first: all you need to know about raw foods. The second: delectable recipes. There's also a *Living on Live Food* DVD (www.alissacohen.com).

Cornbleet, Jennifer. *Raw Food Made Easy for 1 or 2 People.* Summertown, Tenn.: The Book Publishing Co., 2005. A genuinely easy guide to delicious raw food cuisine from a living food chef and educator. (For the companion DVD, go to Cornbleet's site, www.learnrawfood.com.)

Ferrara, Suzanne Alex. *The Raw Food Primer.* Tulsa, Okla., 2003: Council Oaks Books. Artfully presented intro to raw food cuisine from acclaimed live food chef.

Graham, Douglas N., D.C. *The 80/10/10 Diet: Balancing Your Health, Your Weight, and Your Life One Luscious Bite at a Time.* Key Largo, Fla.: FoodnSport Press, 2006. A very low-fat approach to raw foods based on the principles of Natural Hygiene; author has done health coaching for celebs including Martina Navratilova and Demi Moore.

Jones, Susan Smith, Ph.D. *Health Bliss: 50 Revitalizing Super Foods and Lifestyle Choices to Promote Vibrant Health.* Carlsbad, Calif.: Hay House, Inc., 2008. Jones (once told she would never walk again, she's gone on to run races and jump out of airplanes) highlights the fifty most nutritious raw fruits and vegetables, provides dozens of exquisite recipes, and offers positive motivation.

Kenney, Matthew, and Sarma Melngailis. *Raw Food/Real World: 100 Recipes to Get the Glow.* New York: William Morrow, 2005. Exquisite gourmet recipes from the chefs at New York City's five-star raw restaurant, Pure Food and Wine.

HELPFUL RESOURCES, ORGANIZATIONS, AND WEBSITES

*T*he recovery principles in this book can be used to most benefit in a fellowship of individuals recovering in the same fashion. Therefore I heartily recommend:

Overeaters Anonymous, www.overeatersanonymous.org; monthly journal: *Lifeline.* Overeaters Anonymous (OA) uses the Twelve Step program to help people who want to stop eating compulsively. It doesn't endorse any particular plan of eating but deals instead with underlying causes. There's no charge for membership, no weighing at meetings, and no one is too fat or too thin to be welcome. In addition to offering guidance on the Twelve Step way of life, OA provides invaluable peer support and reassurance that you're not alone and that you can recover. Meetings are available around the world; there are also phone and online meetings.

Other sites you may find useful on your weight loss journey include:

www.askthedietitian.com—This site from Joanne Larsen, M.S., R.D., L.D., has the most comprehensive questionnaire/technique for assessing your Body Mass Index (BMI), the fat-to-lean ratio of your body, that I know of. Click on the link for "Healthy Body Calculator."

www.drfuhrman.com—Joel Fuhrman, M.D., is a respected family practitioner and author with an enlightened understanding of weight loss and preventive health.

www.drmcdougall.com—John McDougall, M.D., is a noted internist and an outstanding proponent of a low-fat, plant-based diet; his site provides health information, discussion boards, adventure travel, and a store offering educational materials including the helpful DVD, "Losing Weight without Losing Your Mind," by Douglas Lisle, Ph.D.

www.elasticwaist.com—Elastic Waist is a Condé Nast site about body image, self-acceptance, and being cool with who you are.

www.lovingraw.com—Website and blog for Philip McCluskey, a young man who lost 200 pounds on a raw food diet.

www.nwcr.ws—The National Weight Control Registry is the largest prospective investigation of long-term, successful weight-loss maintenance. It was established in 1994 by Rena Wing, Ph.D., of Brown Medical School, and James O. Hill, Ph.D., of the University of Colorado. If you've maintained a weight loss of thirty pounds or more for at least one year, you can join the study.

www.realage.com—Based on the work of Michael Roizen, M.D., author of *Real Age* and many other books, this site enables you to ascertain your physiological age through a series of questions and provides information for getting physiologically younger.

There are numerous organizations, publications, and sites on the web to help you with your transition to a plant-based diet. Thanks to Mary Max for many of these listings:

www.americanvegan.org—The American Vegan Society, founded in 1960, promotes a vegan diet for individuals and families

www.compassionatecooks.com—Fabulous DVD that shows how to cook and shop cruelty-free

www.earthsave.org—EarthSave International, founded by *Diet for a New America* author John Robbins, promotes a shift toward a healthy, plant-based diet

www.famousveggie.com—Rub elbows (well, cyber-elbows) with the famous www.goveg.com—Info-packed vegan site sponsored by People for the Ethical Treatment of Animals

www.happycow.net—Vegetarian restaurant listings and reviews.

http://navs-online.org—The North American Vegetarian Society, educational organization for promotion of vegetarian ideals; hosts annual conference, Vegetarian Summerfest

www.pcrm.org—Physicians Committee for Responsible Medicine is a group of medical doctors who provide excellent vegetarian nutritional information; they developed the "New Four Food Groups," publish the lay journal *Good Medicine*, and work for alternatives to animal experimentation in medical education and drug and product testing

www.peta.org/accidentallyVegan/—Everyday grocery store food that you never knew was vegan

http://rubies.articledirectoree.com/articles/recipes/non-dairy-cheese-recipes-2_7.html—"Cheese" recipes for cheese lovers

http://store.foodfightgrocery.com—Online vegan grocery store

www.tryveg.com/cfi/toc/?v=07budget—Eating vegan on a budget

www.veganhealth.org—Accurate nutritional info with recommendations regarding specific conditions and situations

www.vegcooking.com—Yummy recipes and general information on vegetarianism

www.vegdining.com—Vegetarian restaurants worldwide

www.vegfamily.com—Info for vegetarian families; includes product reviews and contacts to veg playgroups

www.veggieboards.com—Great information and advice

www.vegnews.com—*VegNews* is a terrific magazine covering every aspect of the vegetarian/vegan diet and lifestyle

www.vegsource.com—Over 10,000 recipes plus discussion boards, articles, experts, newsletter

www.vegsource.com/klaper/index.htm—Michael Klaper, M.D., founder of the Institute of Nutrition Education and Research, offers resources, information, and the opportunity to participate in clinical research on the health status of vegans

www.veggiedate.org—If you're looking for a like-minded love

www.vegpeople.com—Chat, commune, and make friends

www.vegweb.com—Hundreds of reviewed recipes

www.vrg.org—The Vegetarian Resource Group, educational organization with strong nutritional emphasis; site includes recipes, menus, restaurant guide, and online magazine, *The Vegetarian Journal*

CREDITS

In addition to quotations from *Alcoholics Anonymous* (see copyright page), the author gratefully acknowledges permission to quote from:

The Answer to Addiction by John Burns. Copyright 1975. Reprinted by permission of The Queen's Work, Inc.

Nutrition for Vegetarians by Dr. Agatha and Dr. Calvin Thrash. Reprinted by permission of New Lifestyle Books, Seale, Ala.

The Power of Your Plate by Dr. Neal Barnard. Reprinted by permission of The Book Publishing Company, Summertown, Tenn.

Self-Esteem by Virginia Satir. Copyright 1989 by Avanta Network. Reprinted by Permission of Avanta Network.

Sunlight by Zane Kime, M.D. Reprinted by permission of the author.

The Tao of Physics by Fritjof Capra. Copyright 1975, 1983, 1991. Reprinted by arrangement with Shambhala Publications, Inc., Boston.

The Twelve Steps and Twelve Traditions of Overeaters Anonymous by Overeaters Anonymous, Inc. Copyright 1993. Reprinted by permission of Overeaters Anonymous, Inc.

Vegan Nutrition: Pure and Simple by Michael Klaper, M.D. Reprinted by permission of Gentle World.

A Woman Like You by Rachel V. Reprinted by permission of the author.

FOR MORE INSPIRATION

Blog: http://blog.beliefnet.com/yourcharmedlife
Read Victoria's daily blog, "Live Your Charmed Life," in the Holistic Spirituality section of BeliefNet, the web's most comprehensive spirituality site.

Internet radio show: http://www.healthylife.net
To listen to the monthly broadcast, "A Charmed Life," on Creative Health and Spirit Radio, tune in at noon Eastern time on the fourth Friday of every month, or access past programs via the station's archives.

Newsletter: http://www.victoriamoran.com/contact
"The Charmed Monday Minute" goes out to subscribers on a biweekly basis; there is no charge.

Speaking for your business, church, or organization
Victoria's presentations are content-rich, inspiring, funny, and filled with touching and humorous stories your audience won't soon forget. View her speaker demo at www.victoriamoran.com, and read more about her keynotes and workshops on the speaker page of the site. You can then book her directly or be referred to a speakers' bureau that represents her.

Spiritual-life coaching: http:// www.victoriamoran.com/coaching
Victoria is a certified life coach specializing in spiritual-life coaching, i.e., helping you tap the wisdom already inside you to create greater fulfillment, reach your goals, and bring your dreams to fruition.

Web site: http:// www.victoriamoran.com